MANUAL OF CHEST MEDICINE

Already published in the Manuals series

Renal Disease *C. B. Brown*
Clinical Blood Transfusion *M. Brozovic and B. Brozovic*
Haematology *A. S. J. Baughan, A. S. B. Hughes, K. G. Patterson and L. Stirling*
Paediatric Gastroenterology *J. H. Tripp and D. C. A. Candy*

Forthcoming volumes

Cardiology *K. Dawkins*
Gastroenterology *B. T. Cooper and R. E. Berry*
Gynaecology *T. R. Varma*
Infectious Diseases *J. A. Innes*
Neonatal Intensive Care *A. R. Wilkinson*
Rheumatology *J. M. H. Moll*

MANUAL OF CHEST MEDICINE

John E. Stark MA, MD, FRCP
Consultant Thoracic Physician,
Addenbrooke's and Papworth Hospitals,
Cambridge

John M. Shneerson MA, DM, MRCP
Consultant Thoracic Physician,
Addenbrooke's and Papworth Hospitals,
Cambridge and Newmarket General Hospital

Tim Higenbottam BSc, MD, MRCP
Consultant Thoracic Physician,
Addenbrooke's and Papworth Hospitals,
Cambridge

Christopher D. R. Flower MA, FRCP(C), FRCR
Consultant Radiologist,
Addenbrooke's and Papworth Hospitals,
Cambridge

Chapter 34 by
Ben B. Milstein MA, FRCS
Consultant Cardiothoracic Surgeon,
Addenbrooke's and Papworth Hospitals,
Cambridge

Churchill Livingstone
EDINBURGH LONDON MELBOURNE AND NEW YORK 1986

CHURCHILL LIVINGSTONE
Medical Division of Longman Group Limited

Distributed in the United States of America by Churchill Livingstone Inc., 1560 Broadway, New York, N.Y. 10036, and by associated companies, branches and representatives throughout the world.

First published 1986

ISBN   0-443-02737-4

British Library Cataloguing in Publication Data
Manual of chest medicine.
  1. Chest — Diseases
  I. Stark, John E.   II. Milstein, Ben B.
  617'.54   RC941

Library of Congress Cataloging in Publication Data
Manual of chest medicine.
  (Manuals series)
  Includes index.
  1. Chest — Diseases — Handbooks, manuals, etc.
I. Stark, John E. [DNLM: 1. Respiratory Tract
Diseases — handbooks. WF 39 M294]
RC731.M26   1986   617'.54   85–11008

Produced in Longman Singapore Publishers (Pte) Ltd.
Printed in Singapore

Preface

This book is written mainly for doctors in training and is intended to be a straightforward, commonsense and practical guide to diagnosis, investigation and treatment of common respiratory illnesses. It describes the practice of our own unit and therefore concentrates on hospital rather than community problems.

We assume a basic knowledge of terminology, pathology and methods of clinical examination to the level of medical qualifying examinations.

We have not set out to be comprehensive but have given most space to matters which, in our experience, cause difficulty or confusion in the wards and clinics of general hospitals, or where recent ideas or developments have led to differences between the practice of general and thoracic medical departments.

Wherever possible we suggest just one approach to a problem and present alternatives only when these are both widely used in practice (or when we have been unable to agree between ourselves!).

We have aimed for simple colloquial language. Purists may be shocked at our use of 'X-ray' rather than 'radiograph' but this is the term we, and most others, use in day-to-day speech.

We thank our colleagues Ben Milstein for his chapter and Philip Wraight, Don Bethune, Bill Newsom and Nancy Wallis for advice and Rachel Sinfield, Donna Milton and Amanda Brodie for many hours at the word processor.

Cambridge
1986

J. E. Stark
J. M. Shneerson
T. Higenbottam
C. D. R. Flower

Contents

SECTION 1 Some common symptoms and signs   **1**
    1 Breathlessness   3
    2 Cough and sputum   8
    3 Haemoptysis   14
    4 Chest pain   19
    5 Some useful physical signs of generalised lung   23
       disease

SECTION 2 Some methods of investigation   **27**
    6 Radiology of the chest   29
    7 Tests of respiratory function   35
    8 Arterial blood gas analysis   43
    9 Ventilation and perfusion lung scans   47
  10 Bronchoscopy   49
  11 Biopsy of the lung   52
  12 Biopsy of the pleura   54
  13 Transtracheal aspiration   56
  14 Skin tests for atopy   59
  15 Tuberculin skin tests   61

SECTION 3 Some common problems   **65**
  16 Respiratory failure   67
  17 Pulmonary hypertension   77
  18 Pneumonia   82
  19 Lung abscess   89
  20 Lung problems in patients with impaired   93
       respiratory defences
  21 Tuberculosis   99
  22 Bronchiectasis   110
  23 Cystic fibrosis in adolescents and adults   115
  24 Inhaled foreign body   120
  25 Acute thrombo-embolism   123
  26 Pneumothorax   128
  27 Pleural effusion   134
  28 Respiratory problems due to chest wall and   144
       neurological diseases

29 Chronic bronchitis and emphysema   148
30 Asthma   156
31 Lung tumours   173
32 Cryptogenic fibrosing alveolitis and extrinsic   182
    allergic alveolitis
33 Sarcoidosis   187
34 Chest injuries   192
35 Drug-induced lung disease   201
36 Occupation and lung disease   205
37 Pulmonary eosinophilia   213
38 The abnormal chest X-ray   216

SECTION 4   Some aspects of treatment   **227**
39 Oxygen therapy   229
40 Nebulisation of drugs   234
41 Insertion of an intercostal tube   236
42 Endotracheal intubation   239
43 Physiotherapy   243

Index   247

Section 1
SOME COMMON SYMPTOMS AND SIGNS

1. BREATHLESSNESS

Breathlessness (or dyspnoea) is an uncomfortable awareness of breathing. Normal subjects experience breathlessness only during exercise. This sensation increases as maximum rates of work are approached and as maximum rates of exchange of oxygen and carbon dioxide are achieved.

Any disease which limits the exchange of oxygen and carbon dioxide between the tissues and the atmosphere causes more effort to be expended in breathing simply to maintain homeostasis. Increased demand during exercise results in further increase in effort which is perceived as breathlessness. In the most severely afflicted patient this maximum effort of breathing may be present at rest.

SOME GENERAL CAUSES OF BREATHLESSNESS

Lung disease

This leads to disturbance of ventilation and/or perfusion of the lungs.

Chest wall or neurological disease

This reduces ability to ventilate the lungs adequately.

Cardiac disease

The failure of cardiac output to maintain adequate perfusion of exercising muscles leads to anaerobic respiration at low levels of work with resulting metabolic acidosis and breathlessness.

Haematological disease

Anaemia reduces the capacity of blood to carry oxygen

Metabolic disorders

Hyperthyroidism or salicylate poisoning can 'uncouple' the metabolic use of oxygen in tissues resulting in increased 'demand' for oxygen. Acidosis associated with diabetes or renal failure may increase the effort of breathing without altering gas exchange, ventilation being excessive for oxygen needs

Emotional factors

Perception of discomfort, such as pain or breathlessness may be modified by mood. For example patients with chronic lung disease who become depressed may become more breathless simply as a result of a low threshold at which breathlessness is perceived. Some anxious or depressed subjects breathe excessively and may complain not only (or not even) of breathlessness but also of non-respiratory symptoms such as chest pain, light headedness or fatigue ('hyperventilation syndrome').

ASSESSMENT OF THE BREATHLESS PATIENT

The history

How severe is the breathlessness?

Attempt to relate the breathlessness to the rate of performing work. Remember that in adults the maximum capacity for performing work declines with age.

Severity of breathlessness is best graded in descriptive terms, and should be recorded as such in the patients notes, e.g.

— Not breathless except on marked exertion
— Breathless walking up an incline
— Breathless walking on the flat at the same speed as a healthy person of the same age and sex
— Breathless walking on the flat at own pace (record the maximum distance covered)
— Breathless washing, dressing or at rest

How quickly did breathlessness develop?

The speed of development of breathlessness may suggest the cause.

Breathlessness developing within minutes or hours:
— Asthma
— Pulmonary oedema
— Pneumonia
— Pulmonary embolism
— Pneumothorax
— Acute blood loss

Breathlessness developing within days or weeks:
— Cardiac failure
— Pleural effusion
— Thrombo-embolic disease
— Anaemia
— Hyperthyroidism

Breathlessness developing over months or years:
— Chronic obstructive bronchitis
— Emphysema
— Chronic thrombo-embolic disease
— Pulmonary hypertension

What is the pattern and the timing of the breathlessness?
Attacks of breathlessness at night
— Asthma
— Left ventricular failure
— Aspiration of gastro-oesophageal contents
Seasonal breathlessness
— Asthma
Breathlessness lying flat
— Left ventricular failure
— Bilateral diaphragmatic paralysis
— Emphysema (sometimes)
Breathlessness at work or soon after work
— Occupational asthma
— Extrinsic allergic alveolitis
Breathlessness after exercise
— Asthma
Breathlessness at rest
— severe lung disease
— pulmonary oedema
— pulmonary embolism
— functional hyperventilation

What symptoms are present in association with breathlessness?
Wheezing suggests
— Asthma
— Chronic obstructive bronchitis
— Central airway obstruction
Cough suggests
— Chronic obstructive bronchitis
— Asthma
— Pneumonia
— Central airway obstruction
— Pulmonary oedema
— Alveolitis
— Tuberculosis
Pleuritic pain suggests
— Pneumonia
— Pleural effusion
— Pneumothorax
— Pulmonary embolism

Fever suggests
— Pneumonia
— Pulmonary embolism
— Extrinsic alveolitis
Haemoptysis suggests
— Pulmonary embolism
— Bronchial carcinoma
— Tuberculosis
Ankle oedema suggests
— Cor pulmonale
— Pulmonary embolism
Palpitations suggest
— Cardiac disease

What is the social or occupational history?

Cigarette smoking may suggest
— Chronic obstructive bronchitis
— Emphysema
— Bronchial carcinoma
— Ischaemic heart disease
Occupational exposure to inorganic dusts over many years
(e.g. silica, coal dust, asbestos) suggests pneumoconiosis
Exposure to organic dust or chemicals suggests extrinsic
alveolitis, asthma

Any past illnesses?

— Hypertension, myocardial infarction or rheumatic fever
suggest cardiac disease
— Childhood 'bronchitis' suggests asthma or, occasionally,
bronchiectasis
— Pulmonary tuberculosis or severe pneumonia suggests
pulmonary fibrosis or extensive bronchiectasis

Clinical examination

How severe does the breathlessness appear to be?

Record respiratory rate and note whether the patient appears to have
difficulty breathing. A simple test of lung function such as measurements
of PEFR should now be considered an invariable adjunct to physical
examination comparable to measuring the blood pressure.

Any signs of cardiac dysfunction? – Look for

— Tachycardia
— Dysrhythmia
— Hypertension or hypotension
— Third or fourth heart sounds
— Elevated jugular venous pressure
— Ankle oedema
— Late inspiratory crackles

Any signs of diffuse lung disease? (see Chapter 5)
- Wheezing
- Inspiratory crackles (late or early)
- Noisy breathing

Any signs of localised lung disease? – such as
- Consolidation
- Pleural effusion
- Pneumothorax

Clinical investigation

In all patients with breathlessness
1. Chest X-ray (see Chapter 6)
2. Lung function tests (see Chapter 7)
3. Blood count

In selected patients
4. Serum thyroxine
5. Electrocardiogram
6. Arterial blood gas estimation (see Chapter 8).

2. COUGH AND SPUTUM

INTRODUCTION

Cough, one of the commonest symptoms of respiratory disease, has an important function in defence of the lung against inhaled (foreign) material. Both in health and in disease cough may be *involuntary* due to a reflex initiated either by stimulation of the larynx, trachea or larger bronchi, or by loss of compliance of the lung, or it may be a *voluntary* response to awareness of material in the respiratory tract. Cough is considered to be abnormal if it is excessive or inappropriate, or if it produces sputum.

It is important to recognise that failure of the normal coughing mechanism may in itself lead to respiratory disease.
An effective cough requires:
- — A functioning glottis
- — Adequate inspiration and expiration. Either or both may be inadequate if respiratory muscles are paralysed or weak, or if the thoracic cage is deformed
- — Patent airways. Airflow obstruction from any cause impairs expectoration of secretions.
- — Normal bronchial clearance. Mucus may not be cleared effectively from the bronchial tree if its viscosity and elasticity are very abnormal or if there is abnormal ciliary function.

Voluntary and, to a lesser extent, reflex coughing are impaired whenever the level of consciousness is reduced.
An inadequate cough may lead to:
- — Failure to expel material which has been aspirated through the larynx into the lungs such as secretions from the upper respiratory tract, gastro-oesophageal reflux or foreign bodies
- — Accumulation of bronchial secretions.

CLINICAL ASSESSMENT OF COUGH

Listen to the cough. If the glottis is functioning the cough will have a sudden explosive onset. If it is not functioning the initial expiratory noise is less abrupt and is lower pitched ('bovine' cough)

Observe inspiratory and expiratory movements during coughing. An effective cough is impossible without an adequate inspiration

Listen for the sounds produced by secretions. The trained ear can often distinguish between a dry cough, a cough with secretions mainly in the pharynx and a cough with secretions in the lower respiratory tract

Note any hoarseness, stridor or wheeze, which indicate obstruction to larynx, trachea or bronchus, and any abnormalities of phonation or swallowing which might suggest a physical or neurological case for aspiration of liquids or solids into the lungs.

Some causes of dry cough

— Acute inflammation of larynx, trachea and bronchi
— Chronic laryngitis
— Compression of large airways (as by lymph nodes, aortic aneurysm, tumour.)
— Tumour or foreign body in trachea or bronchus
— Asthma
— Pulmonary oedema (of insufficient severity to cause watery sputum)
— Pneumonia (in the early stages)
— Any condition in which the lungs are abnormally stiff, (such as fibrosing alveolitis, sarcoidosis, extrinsic allergic alveolitis)
— Early stages of conditions which later cause sputum (e.g. acute bronchitis)
— Habit.

Sputum

Sputum is the material expectorated from the lower respiratory tract by coughing together with any saliva with which it mixes. The normal bronchial secretions are of insufficient volume to be expectorated, and they are conveyed to the larynx by ciliary action and swallowed. Many patients with increased quantities of sputum do not expectorate because they have adopted the habit of swallowing it. Women and children cough up sputum less often than men for this reason.

Appearance of sputum

This may be an aid to diagnosis but remember that recently swallowed food or drink may contaminate the specimen. Sputum can be differentiated from saliva:

— Saliva usually forms copious clear bubbles on top of any liquid in a sputum pot, which is uncommon with sputum except in pulmonary oedema

— Microscopy of saliva will show squamous cells from the mouth or pharynx, which are absent from bronch-pulmonary secretions.

Appearances

— Mucoid sputum is colourless or white and has a gelatinous consistency. This implies that normal or almost normal mucus is being produced in excessive amounts in the lung or has been inhaled into the bronchial tree. It is commonly produced by patients with simple chronic bronchitis, post-nasal drip asthma or rarely alveolar cell carcinoma

— Plugs of mucus, sometimes branching to form a cast of the bronchial tree, may be coughed up particularly in asthma and allergic broncho-pulmonary aspergillosis

— Purulent sputum is yellow, green or sometimes brown. This implies an inflammatory reaction in the lungs which may be:
   a. infection (purulent bronchitis, pneumonia, lung abscess, bronchiectasis, tuberculosis, cystic fibrosis)
   b. Allergic (sputum of asthmatics may look purulent without any evidence of infection, due to large numbers of eosinophils)
   c. Chemical (acute bronchitis due to inhalation of chemicals)
   d. Irritant (smoke or irritant dusts)

— Watery sputum or pulmonary oedema fluid must be distinguished from saliva (see above)

— Bloody (see Chapter 3)

— Rusty sputum imples a small amount of altered blood mixed with the sputum and occurs particularly in pneumoccal pneumonia and pulmonary oedema

— Solid tissue. Tumour or calcified material (usually pieces of calcified lymph node which have eroded through the bronchial wall) may be expectorated

— Black sputum indicates that carbon is present in large quantities, usually in coal miners with progressive massive fibrosis. Heavy cigarette smokers may produce grey sputum

— 'Anchovy paste' sputum rarely occurs in amoebiasis if necrotic liver is expectorated through a perforation in the diaphragm.

Smell

A strong unpleasant smell suggests anaerobic infection (as from a lung abscess) and this odour may also be apparent on the patient's breath.

Causes of large quantities of sputum

It is important to be sure that all the expectorated material is sputum rather than saliva or material regurgitated from the stomach. It is rare to cough up more than 50 ml of sputum in 24 hours but large volumes may be produced particularly by patients with bronchiectasis, lung abscess, cystic fibrosis or occasionally alveolar cell carcinoma or chronic bronchitis, or with the unusual form of bronchitis associated with ulcerative colitis.

Important points from the history

Has the cough been present for months or years? Suspect chronic bronchitis (productive cough particularly in the morning in a smoker) asthma, bronchiectasis, cystic fibrosis or tuberculosis

Is the cough mainly nocturnal? Suspect asthma, left ventricular failure or aspiration of material into the bronchial tree.

Are there symptoms of laryngeal disease such as hoarse voice?

Are there any symptoms of neurological disease such as coughing whilst eating or drinking, or reflux of fluid through the nose during drinking?

Are there any associated symptoms? Intermittent wheeze suggests asthma. Inspiratory wheeze after paroxysms of cough suggests whooping cough. Fever suggests pneumonia or lung abscess. Haemoptysis suggests carcinoma, tuberculosis or bronchiectasis. Sub-sternal soreness suggests acute tracheitis.

Investigation of cough

Chest X-ray (see Chapter 6)

This may be normal in patients with cough due to:
— Asthma
— Tracheal tumours
— Endobronchial tumours
— Chronic bronchitis
— Bronchiectasis

Sputum microbiology

This is, in practice, rarely of help in diagnosing the cause of cough unless the chest X-ray is abnormal. It may be of diagnostic help in:
— Suspected tuberculosis (see Chapter 21)
— Suspected pneumonia (see Chapter 18)
— Suspected cystic fibrosis (see Chapter 23)

Cytological examination of sputum
This is not recommended as a 'routine' because:
— It is time consuming and expensive
— Failure to see malignant cells does not exclude a diagnosis of cancer
— Bronchoscopy is preferable in most cases if cancer is seriously considered. However if for any reason bronchoscopy is not to be carried out, cytological examination of sputum may confirm, but cannot exclude, a carcinoma (see Chapter 31).

Spirometry
Serial spirometry or records of peak flow may reveal asthma as the cause of a persistent or intermittent cough (see Chapter 30).

Bronchoscopy
This is necessary for all patients with a persistent cough for which no cause has been found, even if the chest X-ray remains normal.

Bronchography
This may, in our experience, reveal previously unsuspected bronchiectasis (see Chapter 22).

Indirect laryngoscopy
This may show a laryngeal cause for cough.

COMPLICATIONS OF COUGH

— Syncope or convulsions are rare and are due to diminished venous return caused by prolonged coughing.
— Vomiting may follow a prolonged bout of coughing particularly in whooping cough, asthma or chronic bronchitis
— Headache is probably due to raised intracranial pressure from impaired venous return during prolonged bouts of coughing
— Chest pain is usually muscular but cough fractures of ribs may occur
— Wheeze. Coughing may induce bronchoconstriction in asthmatics but cough is itself a common symptom of asthma
— Mediastinal emphysema is usually associated with easily recognised supraclavicular subcutaneous emphysema but systolic or diastolic extracardiac clicks or a crunching sound may be heard on auscultation as the only physical sign
— Stress incontinence is common and distressing in multiparous women
— Hernias, inguinal or femoral, may be aggravated by chronic coughing.

TREATMENT OF COUGH

1. Treat the cause whenever possible
2. Suppression of cough is recommended only when there is an exhausting and otherwise untreatable cough – as in some patients with lung cancer. Such coughing may be relieved by:
   Codeine linctus (15 mg in 5 ml)
   Pholcodine linctus strong (10 mg in 5 ml)
   Methadone linctus (2–4 mg in 5–10 ml)
   Remember that these are all also respiratory depressants
3. Bronchodilator drugs such as salbutamol may ease the cough of upper respiratory infections and are best given by inhalation (see Chapter 30)
4. Humidity and warmth may lessen cough as cold, dry air is a potent stimulus to coughing. A warm, humid atmosphere usually suffices but infants with croup may be helped by nebulised saline
5. We do not favour the use of 'mucolytic' agents for treatment of cough
6. Physiotherapy (see Chapter 43).

3. HAEMOPTYSIS

INTRODUCTION

The cause of haemoptysis should always be sought but is frequently not found. It may be difficult to be sure of the source of expectorated blood, particularly if a patient says that he 'just felt the blood in his throat'. It is necessary to consider:
- Blood from nose – does the nose bleed at other times? Did it bleed at the time of the haemoptysis?
- Blood from gums – do gums bleed at other times? Was haemoptysis soon after brushing teeth?
- Blood from throat – was the throat sore or painful at the time of, or before, the haemoptysis?
- Bleeding from the gastro-intestinal tract usually produces brown fluid unless the haemorrhage has been large and very recent.

True haemoptysis is usually followed by blood-streaking of the sputum for a few hours or days. If possible the expectorated material should be seen by the physician, and patients who are no longer producing blood when seen should be asked to save a specimen to bring when they are next seen.

CLINICAL ASSESSMENT

Description of the haemoptysis

- *Repeated small haemoptyses* are often due to bronchial carcinoma, bronchiectasis or pulmonary emboli, and less often to pulmonary hypertension (e.g. mitral stenosis), left ventricular failure or bronchial adenoma, aspergilloma, telangiectasia or intra-alveolar haemorrhage
- *Repeated large haemoptyses* are usually due to chronic inflammatory conditions and the blood is often mixed with pus (bronchiectasis, aspergilloma, lung abscess, tuberculosis). Rarely arterio-venous malformations may cause frequent large

haemoptyses without pus, and bronchial carcinoma can occasionally cause a large haemoptysis
— *Single or infrequent haemoptyses with purulent sputum* may be due to acute bronchitis or to acute exacerbations of chronic bronchitis but such a diagnosis carries a risk as these conditions occur more often in smokers and a bronchial carcinoma may be present. Occasionally pneumonia can cause blood stained sputum but there are usually other features such as fever or breathlessness to suggest an acute infection
— *Single or infrequent haemoptysis without purulent sputum* raises suspicion of bronchial carcinoma especially in cigarette smokers over the age of 40 but pulmonary emboli must be considered. Haemoptysis may follow blunt chest trauma or may occur at the time of a spontaneous pneumothorax. Often, however, no cause is found particularly if the patient is under 40 and is a non-smoker.

Other symptoms

— *Is there pleuritic or chest wall pain*? If so pulmonary emboli, chest trauma or a spontaneous pneumothorax may be the cause
— *Is the patient disproportionately breathless*? Think of pulmonary emboli or a central endobronchial or endotracheal tumour
— *Is the patient wheezy*? Chronic bronchitis should be considered if the wheeze is bilateral and if there is a long history of cough and sputum but unilateral wheeze may be due to bronchial obstruction from carcinoma, adenoma or inhaled foreign body
— *Is there any evidence of heart disease*? Ask about previous rheumatic fever and look for evidence of left ventricular failure, mitral stenosis, pulmonary hypertension or pulmonary emboli
— *Has bleeding occurred at other sites*? If so suspect haemostatic failure.

Examination

— Look for finger clubbing and bruising, and for sources of bleeding in the upper respiratory tract
— Listen for wheeze and note whether it is unilateral or bilateral
— Look for signs of pulmonary consolidation or collapse and for localised inspiratory crackles of bronchiectasis
— Examine the heart carefully and examine the legs for evidence of deep venous thrombosis.

Investigation of haemoptysis

— *A chest X-ray* is essential and both PA and lateral views are required; important abnormalities may be visible only on the lateral views. The chest X-ray may be normal in pulmonary embolism, conditions affecting the larynx, trachea and main bronchi (e.g. adenomas, bronchial carcinoma), primary pulmonary hypertension, bronchiectasis and bronchial telangiectasia.

A normal X-ray makes pulmonary tuberculosis very unlikely but does not exclude a bronchial carcinoma which may produce no radiographic opacity until it is large enough to obstruct a bronchus. Beware a diagnosis of lobar or segmental pneumonia based on X-ray appearances in a patient whose main symptom is haemoptysis. The consolidation may be beyond a bronchial obstruction.

If the X-ray shows evidence of fibrosis and contraction of the upper lobes, previous tuberculosis is a possibility in which case haemoptysis may be due to reactivation of tuberculosis, to development of a mycetoma or to residual bronchiectasis. Previous sarcoidosis may also leave a residue of upper zone fibrosis which may likewise be complicated by mycetoma formation and haemoptysis

— *An electrocardiogram* may rarely give evidence of unsuspected mitral stenosis or of acute or chronic pulmonary hypertension. The ECG is unlikely to be abnormal after a small pulmonary embolism which produced no symptoms other than haemoptysis unless there have been previous episodes resulting in pulmonary hypertension or there is coexistent chronic lung disease

— *Sputum* should be examined microscopically and cultured for tubercle bacilli if there are abnormalities on the chest X-ray compatible with tuberculosis. Cytological examination of sputum following haemoptysis is not recommended as a routine even if bronchial carcinoma is suspected unless bronchoscopy is contraindicated. Failure to detect malignant cells in sputum does not discount a diagnosis of carcinoma and, unless the patient is too ill, too old or is clearly not a candidate for surgical treatment, bronchoscopy is a more certain method of diagnosis

— *Microscopy of urine* for red blood cells which may be present in coagulation defects, generalised vasculitis or Goodpasture's syndrome, which are rare but important cause of haemoptysis

— *Clotting screen and platelet count* if haemostatic failure is suspected from bleeding at several sites or from a bruising tendency

— *Isotope lung scans* (see Chapter 9) are particularly useful if pulmonary embolism is suspected in a patient with a normal chest X-ray. Perfusion scans alone are difficult to interpret if there is pre-existing generalised lung disease, and a ventilation scan is necessary in such patients. Isotope lung scans need not be carried out on all patients with haemoptysis – features such as chest pain, breathlessness, faintness or a predisposing cause will act as a guide

— *Bronchoscopy* carried out immediately after the haemoptysis may enable the site of the bleeding to be identified by tracing the trail of blood down the bronchial tree. More often, however, it is carried out after an interval in a search for an abnormality which may no longer be bleeding. Fibreoptic bronchoscopy is generally preferred but the rigid bronchoscope may be safer after a large haemoptysis as it permits better control of further haemorrhage during the procedure

— *Bronchography* (most conveniently and with least upset to the patient at the time of fibreoptic bronchoscopy) has, in our experience, often revealed unsuspected bronchiectasis in patients who have normal chest X-rays. It is often useful to confirm a suspected diagnosis of bronchiectasis and to delineate its extent, and this is essential if surgical treatment is to be considered.

MANAGEMENT

Emergency treatment for life-threatening haemoptysis

1. Position the patient so that the side of the chest from which the bleeding is probably coming is lowermost, to prevent aspiration of blood into the normal lung and hence prevent drowning
2. Sedate the patient. Diamorphine is the drug of choice
3. Set up an intravenous infusion and collect blood for grouping and possible cross-matching for transfusion
4. Consider endotracheal intubation for aspiration of blood if the patient is at risk of asphyxiating
5. Consider emergency bronchoscopy. The rigid bronchoscope is preferred as it enables blood to be aspirated more easily but bleeding can sometimes be stopped by cold saline lavage through a fibreoptic bronchoscope. A balloon catheter passed through the bronchoscope can be inflated proximally in the bleeding bronchus to isolate the source of the bleeding from the rest of the lung. An experienced bronchoscopist, ideally a

thoracic surgeon, is required for these procedures and should be called before the patient's condition becomes too serious

6. Induction of artificial pneumothorax on the side of the bleeding has been used in an emergency to collapse the lung, lessen its perfusion and reduce bleeding

7. Emergency resection of the lobe or lung which is bleeding may be necessary.

Treatment of smaller haemoptyses

— Haemoptysis itself rarely requires treatment, the aim being to diagnose and treat the underlying condition

— Palliative radiotherapy may stop bleeding in patients with bronchial carcinoma, and bronchial artery embolisation has been used to control haemoptysis in patients with cystic fibrosis

— If no cause is found after investigation, as is commonly the case after a single haemoptysis if the chest X-ray is normal, the patient should be observed with further PA and lateral radiographs for 3–6 months. If the bleeding does not recur and no cause becomes apparent further follow-up is not necessary. All such patients should, however, be advised to report any further haemoptysis or any other respiratory symptoms to their doctor, and in this event further investigation or repetition of previous investigations may be needed to find the cause.

4. CHEST PAIN

Pain arising from each of the major structures within the thorax has distinctive features. The lung itself almost never gives rise to pain.

Trachea

Tracheitis causes a retrosternal soreness or rawness which is worse on inhaling cold air or on coughing. Other tracheal lesions are painless.

Pleura

Visceral pleural disease does not cause pain but pain from the parietal pleura is worse when the two pleural surfaces move rapidly over each other as in coughing, laughing, sneezing, yawning, sighing or taking a deep breath. Other movements of the thorax may also cause pain. The pain is usually sharp and well localised except with a pneumothorax when it may be more diffuse. The pain from the diaphragmatic pleura is referred to the shoulder tip and from the mediastinal pleura may cause pain centrally in the chest or down the inside of the arms.

Pericardium

Pericardial pain is usually substernal but may be felt over a wide area of the thorax. It is often worse when the patient is lying flat and may be exacerbated by inspiration.

Heart

Cardiac pain is usually felt as a heavy or burning pain in the chest and may radiate to the neck (where it may be described as a choking sensation), to the jaw (where it is an ache), into the arms (which feel heavy), or into the fingers (which may feel tingling). Angina is usually related to the degree of exertion or to other factors such as meals, cold weather and emotion. Myocardial infarction causes severe, prolonged pain but of a similar quality to that of angina.

Aorta

Aortic pain from dissection is usually sudden and severe and radiates to the back and shoulders.

Oesophagus

Pain is usually felt in the centre of the chest and may radiate over a wide area and into the arms and neck. It is usually of a burning quality and, if due to gastro-oesophageal reflux, is exacerbated by stooping or lying flat.

Mediastinal lymph nodes

Malignant involvement occasionally causes vague substernal pain.

Nerve roots

Pain radiates round from the spine towards the sternum in an arc corresponding to the appropriate dermatome and is usually worse on movement of the spine but may also be slightly exacerbated by respiratory movements.

Ribs

Rib pain is localised to the site of the abnormality and, particularly if there is a rib fracture, is worse during respiratory movements. Disease of the costochondral junctions is worse on deep inspiration but also causes a well localised continuous ache often with local tenderness on pressure.

HISTORY

- — *How severe is the pain*? Does it stop the patient sleeping and/or working?
- — *Where is the pain most severe* and where does it radiate to? (See above)
- — *How long has the pain been present*? Most patients with pleurisy seek medical advice soon after its onset but non-organic pains may be tolerated for weeks or months before seeking advice
- — *How sudden was the onset of the pain*? It usually starts instantaneously with a pneumothorax, pulmonary embolus, aortic dissection or rupture, myocardial infarction or ruptured oesophagus. Pleuritic pains often come on over a few minutes or some hours
- — *Is the pain affected by movement*, respiratory or other, exertion or food? (see above)

— *What is the quality of the pain?* Pleuritic pains are usually described as 'sharp', cardiac pains as 'heavy' or 'constricting' oesophageal pains as 'burning', tracheal pains as 'sore'. 'Stabbing' pain is very unlikely to have a cardiac or mediastinal origin

— *What relieves the pain?* Is it improved on stopping exertion (suggesting angina), by breathing quietly (suggesting pleurisy) or by alkalis (suggesting oesophagitis)?

— *Are there any associated symptoms?* – such as fever (think of pneumonia, pulmonary embolus), calf pain (think of deep venous thrombosis), cough (think of tracheitis, pneumonia), haemoptysis (think of pulmonary embolism), dyspnoea (think of cardiac disease especially if there is orthopnoea, pulmonary embolism, pneumothorax or pneumonia), acid reflux (think of oesophagitis).

EXAMINATION

— Is there chest wall tenderness to indicate a rib or musculo-skeletal origin of the pain?
— Is there a rash? (herpes zoster)
— Is a pleural or pericardial rub audible?
— Are there signs of a pleural effusion or pericardial effusion?
— Are there signs of cardiac failure, cardiac murmur or 3rd or 4th heart sounds to suggest angina or myocardial infarction?
— Is there radial/femoral artery pulsation delay or any neurological abnormality to suggest aortic dissection?
— Is there peripheral lymphadenopathy which might suggest mediastinal lymph node enlargement as well?
— Is there surgical emphysema in the neck suggesting mediastinal emphysema from a ruptured oesophagus or a pneumothorax?
— Is the pain worse on breathing deeply or on any other movement?
— Are there any neurological signs such as a sensory level or corticospinal tract signs to suggest compression of the thoracic spinal cord?

INVESTIGATIONS

— *A chest X-ray* will show if there is a pleural effusion or pneumothorax, an enlarged heart shadow if there is cardiomegaly or a large pericardial effusion, and may show pneumonia related to pleurisy or the pulmonary, pleural or diaphragmatic changes of a pulmonary embolus (see Chapter 25). It will also show if pulmonary oedema is present in association with cardiac pain. Mediastinal emphysema may not be obvious unless severe. A widened mediastinum may be due to lymph node enlargement, aortic dissection or rarely to a mediastinal tumour which has caused pain by involving the chest wall. A hiatus hernia may be visible behind the heart on both the PA and the lateral film and disease of the thoracic spine should be sought on the lateral view

— *An electrocardiogram* may show left ventricular ischaemia in angina, changes of myocardial infarction, a pattern consistent with a pulmonary embolism, the low voltage complexes due to pericardial effusion or ST elevation and T inversion of pericarditis

— *Barium swallow* may reveal gastro-oesophageal reflux but further investigation, including 24-hour pH monitoring or oesophageal manometry and Bernstein's test, may be required to confirm that this is the cause of the pain

— *Spot X-ray views of the ribs* are better than oblique views for diagnosing rib fractures. If no abnormality is seen a bone scan may be necessary, particularly to confirm metastatic disease

— *Computed tomography* will show mediastinal and some types of pleural disease better than any other technique (see Chapter 6)

— *Lymph node biopsy, arteriography, oesophagoscopy or exercise testing* may be required occasionally to elucidate the nature of chest pain.

TREATMENT

If possible treat the cause of the chest pain rather than the pain itself. Pleuritic and bone pain often responds well to anti-inflammatory analgesics such as indomethacin. Severe pain from a myocardial infarction or aortic dissection requires opiates. If no organic cause is found for the pain reassurance may be effective. Anxiety about the presence of cardiac disease, lung cancer or tuberculosis is a common cause of non-organic chest pain.

5. SOME USEFUL PHYSICAL SIGNS OF GENERALISED LUNG DISEASE

Generalised lung disease (if severe enough to cause any disorder of function) usually results in either generalised airflow obstruction or abnormally stiff lungs, either of which may give rise to diagnostically useful physical signs.

Airflow Obstruction may give rise to wheezes, early inspiratory crackles, noisy breathing or over-inflation.

Wheezes

Wheezes are continuous sounds produced when the walls of partially obstructed airways become opposed and vibrate with the passage of air (analagous to the note made by a reed musical instrument). It is useful to distinguish between 'monophonic' and 'polyphonic' wheezes. A monophonic wheeze equates with a single note from a musical instrument and a polyphonic wheeze with several notes played simultaneously.

A monophonic wheeze implies that a narrowed airway does not vary in calibre during breathing and usually arises from a single narrowed airway. It is a valuable sign of localised narrowing, as from a tumour or stenosis in a bronchus or in the trachea. It may be best or only heard over the site of narrowing.

The much more common polyphonic wheeze is nearly always bilateral and suggests generalised airway narrowing, most often from chronic obstructive bronchitis, emphysema or asthma.

The wheeze of intrathoracic airflow obstruction is predominantly expiratory because the airways, reflecting changes in intrathoracic pressure, tend to widen during inspiration and narrow during expiration.

A predominantly inspiratory wheeze suggests narrowing of the extrathoracic airways (upper trachea or larynx).

Early inspiratory crackles

These discontinuous sounds are heard at the beginning of inspiration and can be audible not only through the stethoscope placed against the chest wall but also when it is held near the patient's open mouth. Early inspiratory crackles are generated by the opening of peripheral airways as lung volume increases during inspiration and indicate severe generalised

airflow obstruction. These crackles may be heard in the absence of
wheeze if airflow obstruction is so severe that there is insufficient flow to
cause the airways to vibrate.

'Noisy Breathing'

These are breath sounds audible without a stethoscope while the patient
is at rest. It is an unmusical sound which is made up of a large number
of frequencies. Noisy breathing is, of course, a normal occurrence during
deep or rapid breathing. Breathing which can be heard from the end of
the bed while a patient breathes at a normal rate at rest suggest severe
airflow obstruction, and occurs in chronic obstructive bronchitis,
emphysema or asthma and with obstruction of the large (central) airways.
A predominantly inspiratory noise is known as stridor and suggests
narrowing of the extrathoracic airway.

Over-inflation

Over-inflation is the result of airflow obstruction and may produce these
non-ausculatory signs:
- Increased resonance on percussion
- Loss of cardiac and hepatic dullness on percussion
- Quiet heart sounds
- Less than 2 finger breadths of trachea palpable above the
  suprasternal notch
- Retraction of the intercostal spaces during inspiration.

The mere shape of the chest (the so called 'barrel-shaped' chest) is not,
in itself, a reliable indication of over-inflation of the lungs and may,
especially in the elderly, merely reflect a thoracic kyphosis.

STIFF LUNGS

Several conditions, most commonly pulmonary oedema, pneumonia or
alveolitis, cause the lungs to become abnormally stiff (reflected
physiologically in a reduction of vital capacity). On auscultation over stiff
lungs crackles can be heard *late* in inspiration and these are thought to
arise from the opening of peripheral airways as the lung volume increases
towards the end of inspiration. Late inspiratory crackles are loudest over
dependent parts of the lungs and therefore 'shift' with alterations in the
patient's position. Unlike the early inspiratory crackles of airflow
obstruction, late inspiratory crackles cannot be heard through the
stethoscope held to the open mouth (Table 5.1).

Table 5.1 Differences between early and late inspiratory crackles

	Early	Late
Vary with posture	No	Yes
Audible at the mouth	Yes	No
Clinical significance	Severe airflow obstruction	Stiff lungs

Section 2
SOME METHODS OF INVESTIGATION

6.   RADIOLOGY OF THE CHEST

STANDARD RADIOGRAPHIC PROCEDURES

The standard chest radiograph

This is normally taken as a posterio-anterior (PA) view with the front of the patient's chest placed against the film cassette. Distortion of intrathoracic structures is reduced by the use of an X-ray tube to film distance of 6 feet or more.

An antero-posterior (AP) view

This may be obtained with the patient's back placed against the film cassette. It is occasionally useful for deciding whether a small opacity on the PA view is genuine by altering its relationship to the overlying rib and unscrambling overlapping vascular shadows. Most AP views, however, are obtained with portable equipment in the ward and the tube to film distance is short. The power of the apparatus is lower and often less consistent than with standard apparatus and the patients under examination are usually ill and difficult to position satisfactorily. The heart and other mediastinal structures may appear unduly large because of the inevitable magnification particularly if the film is exposed with the patient supine. Remember also that both a pneumothorax and free pleural fluid may be difficult to detect with the patient in this position.

The lateral film

This provides a complementary view to the PA.
— It allows one to localise an abnormality seen on the PA view, establish whether opacities occupy the known territory of a lobe or a segment and avoid such catastrophies as mistaking a skin lesion for an intrapulmonary mass
— It provides the best view of the retrosternal and retrocardiac areas and the lung bases
— It may be the only view in which calcification in the aortic and mitral valves is seen.

Over-exposed PA or AP views

Incorrectly termed 'overpenetrated' views, these are obtained by allowing more X-rays to pass through the patient. They are too often used as a substitute for poor quality standard radiography but in centres where high kilovoltage techniques are used for standard radiography (a kVp of 120–140 compared with 60–80) the overexposed view is redundant, for with the high kV technique the mediastinal structures, major airways and spine are all well demonstrated. They are valuable for seeing mediastinal and retrocardiac structures such as the tip of a pacing wire, a mass of sub-carinal nodes, narrowing of a major bronchus or a paravertebral mass.

Oblique projections

These are valuable for demonstrating pleural plaques and other pleural and chest wall lesions in a tangential view.

The apical lordotic view

This is an AP projection obtained with the patient arching his back against the film cassette and is a time-honoured but over-used method of viewing the lung apices. Questionable lesions hidden behind the clavicle may certainly be better seen but lesions above the clavicle are seldom better shown on lordotic views than on the PA projection, and AP tomography is superior for examination of this area.

Decubitus films

These are taken with the patient lying on one side and may be very useful:
— to demonstrate small quantities of pleural fluid and to differentiate between a subpulmonary effusion and a high diaphragm. It is usually better to take these with the affected side lowermost but in the presence of a large effusion, a decubitus film with the affected side uppermost often provides an adequate view of the portion of the lung otherwise obscured by fluid. (Incidentally, this is often a better way of looking at the underlying lung than a chest radiograph following pleural aspiration)
— to demonstrate a small pneumothorax – particularly in severely ill patients.

Films exposed in expiration

These are of value:
— to accentuate a pneumothorax and may indeed be the only means by which a small pneumothorax can be demonstrated

— in any patent suspected of having inhaled a foreign body (the affected lung may exhibit air-trapping remaining larger and more transradiant than its counterpart)
— if partial central airway occlusion by tumour is suspected, when there may also be air-trapping on an expiratory film
— in Macleod's syndrome.

Fluoroscopy ('screening')

— This is of value to assess diaphragmatic function but may be misleading if both diaphragmatic leaves are paralysed
— Fluoroscopy has been largely superceded by ultrasound and computed tomography in patients suspected of having a subphrenic abscess
— It is unreliable for the differentiation of a mediastinal aneurysm from a solid mass because distinction between the intrinsic pulsation of an aneurysm and the transmitted pulsation from a solid lesion is extremely difficult.

Barium swallow

This is valuable:
— to demonstrate oesophageal lesions which may be responsible for pulmonary disease (gastro-oesophageal reflux, achalasia, a vascular ring, posterior oesophageal pouch)
— occasionally, for the indirect assessment of masses in the middle and posterior mediastinum.

READING THE CHEST RADIOGRAPH

Chest films are the most common radiographic examinations and are amongst the most difficult to interpret.
1. View a film with an orderly search pattern
2. In the light of the clinical problem consider carefully what to look for, rather than what to look at. The following hints may prove useful:
   a. *Examine any previous films* in sequence, ideally on a large screen so that they can be viewed together and compared. This will reveal whether an opacity is recent and will also show the rate of change
   b. *Note poor radiographic technique* such as rotation or poor inspiration which may, for example, make the normal heart, mediastinum or lungs appear abnormal
   c. *Check the patient's name and date of the radiograph*

    d. *If the radiograph looks normal* look again:
- (i) behind the clavicles
- (ii) through the heart at the lung bases and medial parts of the lower lobes
- (iii) just above the diaphragms for abnormal shadowing
- (iv) at the size, shape, density and position of the hila (the left hilum is normally slightly higher than the right – but should be of equal density and size)
- (v) the lungs are normally equally transradiant and any discrepancy must be explained.

3. On the lateral film check:
   a. are the retrosternal and retrocardiac triangles of equal transradiancy?
   b. Are the thoracic vertebral bodies, as they should be, darker the more caudal they are?
   c. are the posterior costophrenic angles sharp?
   d. are both diaphragmatic leaves well-defined?
4. If the heart or mediastinum look abnormal check if the film was exposed with the patient supine or rotated either of which may cause apparent deformity of a normal mediastinum.

Pre-operative chest radiographs

These are necessary for patients before elective (non-cardiopulmonary) surgery if:
- the patient has cardiac or respiratory symptoms
- the patient has cancer and demonstration of pulmonary metastases will influence management
- the patient is an immigrant from a country where tuberculosis is still endemic.

Views differ as to whether or not routine chest X-rays should be taken on all patients over the age of 45 prior to major surgery. Such films would be justified only if an incidental finding would influence management.

SPECIALISED TECHNIQUES

Conventional tomograms

These are obtained by the synchronous movement of film-holder and X-ray tube which produces blurring of all but one plane of the structures filmed. They are useful:
- to confirm and define a suspected hilar mass (oblique and lateral projections are the best)

— to confirm and define suspected disease at the apex of the lung
— to confirm and define a possible pulmonary opacity on the plain chest radiograph
— to show certain important characterisatics of a solitary pulmonary mass (central calcification in a granuloma, air to indicate cavitation, feeding vessels to indicate an arterio-venous malformation)
— to demonstrate small pulmonary metastases which are not visible on standard films
— to confirm and define a suspected mediastinal mass.

Computed tomography (CT)

CT has superceded conventional tomography in many instances – particularly in cases 5 & 6 above. Its main uses are:
— to assess the mediastinum. C.T. resolves the problem of the questionably abnormal mediastinum, accurately localises mediastinal masses and may sometimes yield a definite diagnosis as for example of an aneurysm or of a fluid or fat-containing tumour
— to demonstrate and localise pleural disease
— to demonstrate pulmonary or mediastinal metastases
— to stage tumours
— to demonstrate pulmonary disease in the presence of a pleural effusion
— to demonstrate subphrenic disease, such as abscess
— to show whether any intrathoracic disease is present when a questionable abnormality is suspected on plain radiographs.

Radionuclide imaging (see Chapter 9)

Pulmonary angiography

This is performed by injection of contrast medium into the main pulmonary artery or one of its major branches through a catheter passed under fluoroscopic control through the heart from an antecubital or femoral vein. Its main uses are:
— to demonstrate pulmonary emboli. Radionuclide imaging has greatly reduced the need for pulmonary angiography for diagnosis of pulmonary embolism, but it is required when patients are suspected of having had a massive embolus, in those with suspected pulmonary embolism where the radionuclide scans are equivocal, and if thrombolytic therapy is to be given (see Chapter 25)
— to demonstrate pulmonary arterio-venous malformation
— to demonstrate some other congenital pulmonary abnormalities (such as pulmonary atresia).

Bronchography

This technique is used much less now than in the past because of the decline in the prevalence and surgical treatment of bronchiectasis. When required it is now ideally performed via the fibreoptic bronchoscope except in children when a general anaesthetic is necessary. The main indication remains the demonstration or exclusion of bronchiectasis (See Chapter 22).

Ultrasound

This has become increasingly valuable in the diagnosis and management of pleural disease and also of subphrenic infection. Either A mode or real time techniques can be used. It provides a simple and reasonably reliable technique for distinguishing between pleural fluid and pleural thickening or tumour – a distinction which is not always apparent from physical examination of the chest or from the radiograph. With ultrasound the exact site of fluid can be determined before aspiration, which is particularly useful when the fluid is loculated or small in quantity.

Lung biopsy

See Chapter 11 for biopsy techniques some of which require X-ray visualisation of the lung or of the opacity to be biopsied.

7. TESTS OF RESPIRATORY FUNCTION

Uses of pulmonary function tests

— To identify or exclude a respiratory cause of breathlessness
— To identify the type of impairment of respiratory function as an aid to diagnosis
— To quantify any disturbance of lung function.

WIDELY AVAILABLE TESTS

Peak expiratory flow rate (PEFR)

Equipment
Either a robust metal peak flow meter or lighter and cheaper plastic meters are available.

Method
The patient inhales fully, then forcibly exhales into a peak expiratory flow meter which records the highest flow rate attained. The result is usually expressed as l/min.

Problems with use
— Failure to exhale with maximal force.
— Failure to seal the mouth around the mouth piece (inadvertently or due to facial weakness)
— Failure to inhale fully before blowing.

Interpretation
Predicted value for normal subjects are shown in Table 7.1. Values less than 80% of predicted are abnormal).
— The PEFR is reduced in airflow obstruction, as in asthma, chronic obstructive bronchitis or emphysema
— PEFR may be reduced in patients who have respiratory muscle weakness
— PEFR may be normal or even increased in patients with pulmonary fibrosis.

Table 7.1 Predicted normal values for PEFR (litres/min)

height						age				
	25	30	35	40	45	50	55	60	65	70
MALES										
5'3"	572	560	548	536	524	512	500	488	476	464
5'6"	597	584	572	559	547	534	522	509	496	484
5'9"	625	612	599	586	573	560	547	533	520	507
6'0"	654	640	626	613	599	585	572	558	544	530
6'3"	679	665	650	636	622	608	593	579	565	551
FEMALES										
4'9"	377	366	356	345	335	324	314	303	293	282
5'0"	403	392	382	371	361	350	340	329	319	308
5'3"	433	422	412	401	391	380	370	359	349	338
5'6"	459	448	438	427	417	406	396	385	375	364
5'9"	489	478	468	457	447	436	426	415	405	394

Standard Deviation = 60 (litres/min)
Ethnic differences negligible
Data derived from Cotes J E 1978 Lung Function, 4th edn. Blackwell, Oxford

Forced expired volume in 1 second (FEV1) and vital capacity (VC)

These are usually measured with a dry wedge spirometer (Vitalograph) but other equipment is available.

Method

The patient inhales fully then forcibly exhales into the mouth piece until no more air can be expelled. A chart records volume exhaled against time from which both the FEV_1 and FVC (forced vital capacity) can be measured (Fig. 7.1). It may be an advantage to record the 'relaxed' VC separately by asking the patient to make a full but unhurried exhalation into the spirometer.

Problems with use

These are the same as PEFR. The measurement of VC is open to error in patients with severe lung disease who are unable to hold their breath for long enough to exhale fully or who cough during the manoeuvre. Patients may not maintain their expiratory effort throughout the test; this is apparent on inspection of the tracings which show an irregular or wavy rather than a smooth line.

Interpretation

Predicted values of FEV_1 and FVC for normal subjects are shown in Tables 7.2 & 7.3. Values less than 80% of predicted are definitely abnormal.

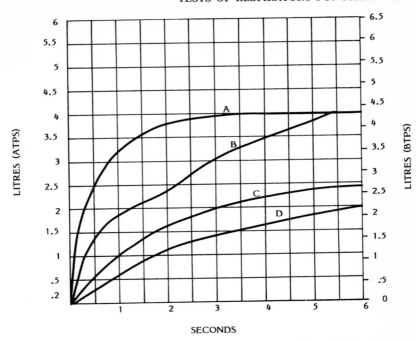

Fig. 7.1 The Spirogram (Dry Spirometer – 'Vitalograph'): A. normal; B. technically unsatisfactory as the patient has not sustained a forced experation; C. airflow obstruction; D. airflow obstruction – vital capacity has been under-estimated as the line would have continued to rise after 6 seconds.

Table. 7.2 Predicted normal values for FEV_1 (litres)

height	age									
	25	30	35	40	45	50	55	60	65	70
MALES										
5'3"	3.61	3.45	3.30	3.14	2.99	2.83	2.68	2.52	2.37	2.21
5'6"	3.86	3.71	3.55	3.40	3.24	3.09	2.93	2.78	2.62	2.47
5'9"	4.15	4.00	3.84	3.69	3.53	3.38	3.22	3.06	2.91	2.75
6'0"	4.44	4.28	4.13	3.97	3.82	3.66	3.51	3.35	3.20	3.04
6'3"	4.69	4.54	4.38	4.23	4.07	3.92	3.76	3.61	3.45	3.30
FEMALES										
4'9"	2.60	2.45	2.30	2.15	2.00	1.85	1.70	1.55	1.40	1.25
5'0"	2.83	2.68	2.53	2.38	2.23	2.08	1.93	1.78	1.63	1.48
5'3"	3.09	2.94	2.79	2.64	2.49	2.34	2.19	2.04	1.89	1.74
5'6"	3.36	3.21	3.06	2.91	2.76	2.61	2.46	2.31	2.16	2.01
5'9"	3.59	3.44	3.29	3.14	2.99	2.84	2.69	2.54	2.39	2.24

Standard Deviation = (Males) 0.5 litres; (Females) 0.4 litres
Ethnic Factor = −0.4 litres
Data derived from Cotes J E 1978 Lung Function, 4th edn. Blackwell, Oxford

Table 7.3 Predicted normal values for FVC (litres)

height					age					
	25	30	35	40	45	50	55	60	65	70
MALES										
5'3"	4.17	4.06	3.95	3.84	3.73	3.62	3.51	3.40	3.29	3.18
5'6"	4.53	4.42	4.31	4.20	4.09	3.98	3.87	3.76	3.65	3.54
5'9"	4.95	4.84	4.73	4.62	4.51	4.40	4.29	4.18	4.07	3.96
6'0"	5.37	5.26	5.15	5.04	4.93	4.82	4.71	4.60	4.49	4.38
6'3"	5.73	5.62	5.51	5.40	5.29	5.18	5.07	4.96	4.85	4.74
FEMALES										
4'9"	3.13	2.98	2.83	2.68	2.53	2.38	2.23	2.08	1.93	1.78
5'0"	3.45	3.30	3.15	3.00	2.85	2.70	2.55	2.40	2.25	2.10
5'3"	3.83	3.68	3.53	3.38	3.23	3.08	2.93	2.78	2.63	2.48
5'6"	4.20	4.05	3.90	3.75	3.60	3.45	3.30	3.15	3.00	2.85
5'9"	4.53	4.38	4.23	4.08	3.93	3.78	3.63	3.48	3.33	3.18

Standard Deviation = (Males) 0.6 litres; (Females) 0.4 litres
Ethnic Factor = (Males) −0.7 litres; (Females) −0.6 litres
Data derived from Cotes J E 1978 Lung Function, 4th edn. Blackwell, Oxford

— The FEV_1 is reduced in patients with airflow obstruction. The VC may also be reduced, but less so than the FEV_1, so the ratio FEV_1/VC (forced expired ratio or FER) normally greater than 75% is reduced
— Both FEV_1 and VC are reduced when the lungs are of small volume (lung fibrosis, pulmonary oedema), when the respiratory muscles are weak or when the chest wall is diseased. The FER is therefore normal
— In patients with emphysema the forced vital capacity may be considerably lower than the relaxed VC, so the latter measurement is preferable.

Carbon monoxide gas transfer (TLCO) (Diffusing capacity of the lung)

Method
This is normally measured with an automated device available only in a respiratory laboratory. The patient inhales fully from residual volume (RV) a mixture of air, helium and carbon monoxide, holds the breath for 10 seconds and exhales slowly. During the exhalation a sample of the expired air is collected and is analysed for helium and carbon monoxide content. Knowing the initial concentrations of the inhaled gases, as helium is inert and is not absorbed the dilution of helium allows the volume of distribution of the gas mixture to be calculated. This is called the alveolar gas volume (Va). Carbon monoxide on the other hand

rapidly combines with alveolar capillary blood to give
carboxyhaemoglobin. The rate of transfer of carbon monoxide depends
upon the volume of blood coming into contact with the inhaled gases
which, in turn, depends on the pulmonary capillary blood volume and the
distribution of ventilation and perfusion in the lungs. TLCO is expressed
as the uptake of CO per minute per unit partial pressure gradient of CO
(mmol/min KPa), or as the transfer coefficient (KCO) which is the
TLCO per litre of alveolar air.

Problems in use

It is not possible to measure TLCO by this method in patients who:
- are too breathless to hold their breath for 10 seconds. This
  usually applies to patients with VC below 1 litre
- are unable for any reason to coordinate their breathing to
  inhale fully, hold their breath, then exhale.

Interpretation

A low TLCO may result from:
- reduction of the number of alveolar capillaries (as in
  emphysema, pulmonary fibrosis or pulmonary emboli)
- disturbance of the normal matching of ventilation and
  perfusion (as in oedema, exudate or infiltrate)
- reduced amount of haemoglobin in blood (anaemia).

A high TLCO may occur:
- physiologically during exercise
- in asthma (probably as a result of redistribution of blood
  within the pulmonary circulation)
- in alveolar haemorrhage
- in polycythaemia.

The results of TLCO measurements should not be interpreted in isolation
but in relation to spirometry and, if available, with measurements of total
lung capacity (TLC).

LESS WIDELY AVAILABLE TESTS

Total lung capacity (TLC), residual volume (RV) and functional residual volume (FRC)

Methods

There are a number of methods of measuring TLC, RV and FRC
including whole body plethysmography, helium re-breathing (using the
equipment for measuring gas transfer) and computing volumes from
posterior-anterior and lateral chest radiographs.

Interpretation

TLC is increased in emphysema and asthma but is reduced when the
lungs are 'stiff' as in pulmonary fibrosis or pulmonary oedema, and in
disorders of the chest wall or respiratory muscles.

RV is increased in chronic obstructive bronchitis, emphysema and asthma and is decreased when the lungs are small or 'stiff'.

FRC is increased in the presence of airflow obstruction and decreased in patients with 'stiff' or small lungs and with chest wall deformity or neurological diseases affecting respiratory muslces.

Flow volume loop (FV curve)

Methods
The patient inhales fully then exhales forcefully into a device which simultaneously records expiratory flow and exhaled volume. On reaching residual volume (RV) the patient then rapidly inhales again to TLC. Flow and volume are displayed graphically.

Interpretation
The flow volume loop has proved valuable in distinguishing intrathoracic from extrathoracic airflow obstruction. Narrowing of the airway outside the thorax (in the upper trachea or larynx) causes predominant obstruction during inspiration whereas intrathoracic obstruction limits expiration. The flow volume loop is a sensitive method of detecting these differences.

Airway resistance (Raw)

Method
This measurement is made using a whole body plethysmograph.

Interpretation
Raw is increased in airway obstruction, (chronic obstructive bronchitis, emphysema, asthma or intra- and extra-thoracic central airway obstruction). Raw is not increased in patients with respiratory muscle weakness.

TESTS OF EXERCISE TOLERANCE

It is sometimes valuable to measure exercise tolerance, either for assessment of disability or to measure the response to therapy.

Simple tests

Corridor walking distance
The patient is asked to walk as quickly as possible along a level corridor, taking as many rests as are needed. The distance covered in 6 or 12 minutes (including the time for stops) is recorded as a simple test of exercise tolerance. It is mainly of use in patients with severe respiratory disability.

Table 7.4 Some patterns of lung function changes in common diseases

	Pulmonary fibrosis or oedema	Chest wall or neuromuscular disease	Emphysema	Chronic obstructive bronchitis	Asthma	Anaemia, pulmonary embolism
PEFR	N	↓	↓	↓	↓	N
FEVI	↓	↓	↓	↓	↓	N
VC	↓	↓	↓	↓	↓	N
FEVI/VC	N	N	↓	↓	↓	N
TLCO & KCO	↓	↓ (KCO↑)	↓	N	N or ↑	↓
TLC	↓	↓	↑	↑	↑	N
RV	↓	↓	↑	↑	↑	N
RV/TLC	N	↑	↑	↑	↑	N

N = Normal; ↑ = Increased; ↓ = Decreased

Complex tests

These are available in specialised laboratories where rate of oxygen consumption and of CO_2 production, minute ventilation, tidal volume, respiratory rate and heart rate are recorded during progressively increasing work on either a cycle ergometer or a mechanical treadmill. Their main value is:

— To distinguish between cardiac and pulmonary causes of breathlessness

— To establish the severity of respiratory and/or cardiac disease

— To establish if any respiratory or cardiac disease is present in, for example, a breathless patient in whom no abnormality has been found on clinical examination, X-ray and other tests.

The patterns of lung function changes usually seen in common diseases are summarised in Table 7.4. These are considered in more detail in the relevant chapters.

8. ARTERIAL BLOOD GAS ANALYSIS

Most hospitals now have automated equipment for analysis of arterial blood to provide values for:
- Oxygen tension (Pao_2)
- Carbon dioxide tension ($Paco_2$)
- Oxygen saturation
- pH (or hydrogen ion concentration)
- Base excess or bicarbonate concentration

The methods of analysis used will not be described here but the inportance of careful calibration of equipment must not be forgotten especially when measurements are carried out by medical rather than technical staff.

SAMPLING ARTERIAL BLOOD

1. The prefered site for obtaining a sample of arterial blood is the brachial artery which is found by palpating the medial part of the antecubital fossa. The radial artery is palpated at the wrist and the femoral artery in the groin. The small size of the radial artery and the greater risk of infection or leakage at the femoral artery make these less desirable sites for sampling
2. Prepare a 5 ml syringe by drawing up a small amount of heparin (1000 units/ml) and expelling it through a needle. This leaves the barrel of the needle filled with heparin to prevent clotting of the sample but the small volume of dilute heparin has no significant effect upon the pH of the sample
3. The skin overlying the puncture site may if needed be anaesthetised with 1% lignocaine but this is usually unnecessary
4. Identify the site of arterial puncture with the left index finger and insert the needle, at an angle of 45 degrees to horizontal, towards the artery. On entering the artery blood will usually pulsate into the syringe or will readily enter the barrel on withdrawing the plunger. Unless the patient is very hypoxic the bright colour of arterial blood is obvious

5. Collect 4–5 ml and remove the needle from the artery immediately applying firm pressure over the puncture site. Pressure should be maintained for 4 minutes (or longer if the patient has a bleeding tendency)
6. Immediately expel any air from the syringe, which must then be capped with an airtight seal
7. The sample must be taken immediately for analysis. If there is to be any delay the syringe should be immersed in iced water. Expulsion of air, sealing the syringe, speed of analysis and cooling of the specimen are all precautions against further changes in oxygen or CO_2 content either from equilibration with air or from metabolic processes in the blood
8. Observe the puncture site for haematoma and check for normal arterial pulsation distal to the puncture site.

Repeated arterial blood analysis

In the critically ill patient repeated sampling of arterial blood may be necessary and to avoid repeated punctures, which are painful and risk damage to the artery, an indwelling arterial catheter can be inserted.

A specially designed arterial cannula is inserted, usually into the radial artery, and clotting is prevented by an infusion of dilute heparin saline at a very slow rate.

USES OF ARTERIAL GAS ANALYSIS

— For diagnosis and assessment of respiratory failure of any type by measurement of Pa_{O_2} and Pa_{CO_2} (see Chapter 16)
— For assessing the response to oxygen therapy (see Chapter 38)
— For assessing acid-base balance. The lungs excrete over 100 times more acid (as carbon dioxide) than do the kidneys. The pH (hydrogen ion content) of arterial blood is determined by the reaction between carbon dioxide and water of the blood:

$$CO_2 + H_2O \rightleftharpoons H_2CO_3 \leftrightharpoons H^+ + HCO_3$$

This reaction may be expressed:
pH = pKa + log $(HCO_3/P_{CO_2} + 0.03)$
pKa is a constant of value 6.1 so that if the ratio $(HCO_3/P_{CO_2} + 0.030)$ is equal to 20
pH = 6.1 + log 20 = 7.4 (or hydrogen ion concentration = 40 nmol/l).

Bicarbonate concentration is determined mainly by the kidneys and P_{CO_2} by the lungs. An excess of bicarbonate ions above normal can be expressed as the 'base excess'.
— For quantifying right to left intracardiac shunts.

Abnormalities of acid-base balance

Respiratory acidosis

This results from an increase of $P\text{CO}_2$ which reduces the ratio ($HCO_3/P\text{CO}_2$ + 0.030) leading to a fall of pH (or rise of H^+ concentration).

$P\text{CO}_2$ rises when, as a result of inadequate ventilation, CO_2 loss from the lungs is reduced relative to metabolic production of CO_2. The causes are discussed in Chapter 16.

If respiratory acidosis persists renal compensation occurs by excretion of a more acid urine and tubular retention of bicarbonate ions. Plasma HCO_3 rises and the ratio ($HCO_3/P\text{CO}_2$ + 0.03) approaches normal, restoring pH (or H^+ concentration). The increased plasma bicarbonate may be expressed as a 'Base Excess' i.e. the excess of bicarbonate ions above normal.

Impaired renal tubular function may reduce reabsorption of bicarbonate and hence prevent compensation of respiratory acidosis. A persistently low pH is a bad prognostic sign in patients with acute respiratory acidosis.

Respiratory alkalosis

This can result from a fall of $P\text{CO}_2$ which increases the ratio ($HCO_3/P\text{CO}_2$ + 0.03) and thereby raises pH (reduces H^+ concentration). Such a fall of P_{CO_2} results from over ventilation from any cause. It is seen in many patients with the conditions causing acute hypoxic respiratory failure (see Chapter 16) or during voluntary or emotional hyperventilation.

Renal compensation may occur through increased tubular excretion of bicarbonate ions (reducing the ratio ($HCO_3/P\text{CO}_2$ + 0.03) towards normal). This is reflected in a fall of plasma bicarbonate or a base deficit ('negative base excess').

Metabolic acidosis

This occurs as a result of a fall of HCO_3 due to accumulation of acid in the blood. The ratio ($HCO_3/P\text{CO}_2$ + 0.03) thereby falls.

Common causes are renal failure, diabetic ketoacidosis or salicylate overdosage, but severe metabolic acidosis may also occur in shock (circulatory collapse) when tissue hypoxia leads to accumulation of lactic acid.

Compensation is respiratory with an increase in ventilation which causes a fall of $P\text{CO}_2$. Hence in this situation there is a reduced $P\text{CO}_2$ together with a reduced bicarbonate (base deficit; 'negative base excess').

Metabolic alkalosis

This results from a rise of HCO_3 which elevates the ratio ($HCO_3/P\text{CO}_2$ + 0.03). This may follow ingestion of alkalis, severe or prolonged vomiting or potassium depletion.

Respiratory compensation takes the form of reduced ventilation causing a rise of $P\text{CO}_2$. In this situation an elevated $P\text{CO}_2$ is associated with a raised bicarbonate concentration (base excess). This is therefore an important, but uncommon, distinction from the more common respiratory acidosis of respiratory failure.

Note: Respiratory and metabolic disturbances frequently occur together, complicating interpretation of blood gas analysis. For example, in acute hypoxic respiratory failure which is complicated by cardiogenic shock (as in severe pulmonary oedema) respiratory alkalosis resulting from over ventilation may be accompanied by a metabolic acidosis due to release of lactic acid from hypoxic tissues.

9. VENTILATION AND PERFUSION LUNG SCANS

Isotope lung scanning offers a means of studying the distribution of ventilation and perfusion in different regions of the lungs. It depends upon the principle of delivering a gamma ray emitting nuclide (isotope) to the alveoli for ventilation and to the pulmonary capillaries for perfusion.

Ventilation scans

Ventilation scans may be obtained using different isotopes.

— An aerosol of a solution in saline of technetium-99m chelated to DTPA (Diethylene-triamine-penta-acetate) is nebulised to give particles of less than 1 micron in size which are inhaled during quiet breathing. The material for the scan can be kept available in any hospital but a special nebuliser is required. Because a ventilation scan must be performed before a perfusion scan, a decision about the need for a ventilation scan must be made at the outset

— Krypton-81m with a half-life of only 13 seconds can be inhaled during tidal breathing to provide an image of ventilation. As the energy level of the gamma emission is different from technetium-99m ventilation images can be obtained after the perfusion image has been reviewed. However the isotope is obtained from a cyclotron, is very expensive, and can be obtained only on certain days by special arrangement with a cyclotron unit

— The long half-life gas xenon-133 may be used to determine regional ventilation but requires patients to co-operate, breathing from a spirometer while the wash-in and wash-out of the isotope is recorded. The method is therefore not suitable for a very ill or breathless patient. Although xenon is readily available, a computer or microprocessor on line to the gamma camera is required to obtain a ventilation image if this is performed after the perfusion scan or if functional information is required.

Perfusion scans

Perfusion scans are obtained by intravenous injection of microparticles of albumin labelled with technetium-99m. These particles range from 15 to 70 microns in diameter and, being of similar density to red blood cells, are distributed in the pulmonary circulation in proportion to regional blood flow. Because of their size they impact in pulmonary capillaries, but as the number of particles is small compared with the number of pulmonary arterioles haemodynamic effects from obstruction of the pulmonary vascular bed are very rare.

Imaging
Six views of the lungs are obtained by positioning the patients in front of a gamma camera to obtain anterior, posterior, right and left lateral as well as right and left posterior oblique views. This provides anatomical information so that 'defects' in lobar or segmental perfusion or ventilation may be detected. Using xenon, only one view can be obtained.

Clinical uses of lung scans

The major use is in the diagnosis of suspected pulmonary embolism (see Chapter 25).

— In patients with no other respiratory illness and with a normal chest radiograph multiple segmental defects of perfusion indicate a high probability of pulmonary emboli

— Difficulties of interpretation arise however, in patients with lung diseases which alter ventilation, for example pneumonia, pulmonary fibrosis, asthma, emphysema and chronic obstructive bronchitis, because local perfusion may be impaired secondarily to ventilation. In patients with any of these conditions therefore, both perfusion and ventilation scans should be performed because defects of perfusion may be due to the underlying lung disease and are therefore not specific for emboli. In such patients perfusion defects which are normally ventilated strongly favour pulmonary emboli, but matched defects of ventilation and perfusion may be due to underlying disease. It is important to recognise, however, that even matched defects of perfusion and ventilation may be caused by emboli and this finding does not therefore exclude this diagnosis.

Safety
Perfusion and ventilation scans are extremely safe procedures and, in spite of earlier fears, we know of no proven risks of the procedure in patients with pulmonary hypertension or intracardiac shunts.

10. BRONCHOSCOPY

Since the introduction of the flexible fibreoptic bronchoscope there has been a great increase in the scope of endoscopic examination of patients with a wide range of pulmonary disorders. Unlike rigid bronchoscopy which requires general anaesthesia, fibreoptic bronchoscopy requires no more than pre-medication and topically applied local anaesthetic. The procedure can be carried out in a side-room, in an X-ray suite or in the ward.

The fibreoptic bronchoscope can be used to:
- Examine the bronchial tree to view and biopsy lesions within the lumen, or involving the wall of the trachea or bronchi
- Biopsy the substance of the lung (transbronchial biopsy) or the bronchial mucosa
- Remove secretions from the bronchial tree either for laboratory examination or as a form of treatment
- Wash out small bronchi and alveoli to sample cells for laboratory examination (broncho-alveolar lavage)
- Aspirate cellular material from masses which are outside the bronchial tree
- Deliver contrast medium to obtain a bronchogram (see Chapter 6).

Indications

- Haemoptysis (see Chapter 3)
- Unresolved, or incompletely resolved, pneumonia (see Chapter 18)
- Certain pulmonary opacities seen on the chest X-ray (see Chapter 38)
- Diffuse lung shadowing (see Chapter 38)
- Infections when sputum cannot be obtained or when sputum examination may be misleading beacuse of upper respiratory tract contamination
- Bronchiectasis, by providing a route for bronchography
- Treatment of severely ill patients with excessive secretions in the airway which cannot be removed by coughing or other methods of suction.

Fibreoptic bronchoscopy usually takes about 30 minutes. Most patients are able to return home 4 hours after bronchoscopy but should not drive a car on the same day if they have received any sedative drugs. We prefer those who have had lung biopsy or bronchography to remain under observation in hospital for 24 hours.

Preparation of the patient

1. The procedure should be fully explained to the patient and his signed consent obtained. The procedure should not be painful but patients may cough and have a transient awareness of an obstruction to breathing while the bronchoscope is being passed
2. Food and drink is witheld for 4 hours before endoscopy
3. Pre-medication varies at different centres. We given omnopon and scopalomine (analgesic plus anticholinergic) intramuscularly one hour before the procedure. An adult of normal build receives 15 mg omnopon with 0.3 mg scopolomine but the dose can be increased to 20 mg and 0.4 mg respectively for an apprehensive patient. Omnopon carries a risk of producing respiratory depression.

   Patients with an FEV_1 of under 1 litre should have arterial blood gases measured before bronchoscopy. If arterial P_{CO_2} is raised the need for bronchoscopy should be carefully reconsidered, but if it is decided to proceed the dose of omnopon should be reduced to half the usual dose or even omitted. Such a patient should be carefully observed during and after bronchoscopy for evidence of worsening respiratory failure and, if this occurs, naloxone (0.4 mg) should be given I.M. or I.V. Hypoxia may worsen during bronchoscopy and oxygen should be given during bronchoscopy if the initial arterial P_{O_2} is less than 6.5 Kpa. If there is also elevation of P_{CO_2} the usual precautions for oxygen therapy are necessary (see Chapter 16)
4. Patients must not drink or eat for 4 hours after the procedure because of the risk of inhaling food through an anaesthetised larynx.

The procedure

The patient can recline on pillows or lie flat. Lignocaine spray or gel is instilled into one nostril. The bronchoscope is lubricated and then inserted through the nostril to a position above the larynx. 2% lignocaine is then instilled down the suction channel of the bronchoscope onto the larynx which is carefully examined. The bronchoscope is then passed through the vocal cords into the trachea. More lignocaine is delivered as the trachea, main bronchi, lobar and segmental bronchi are examined in turn. A good view should be obtained of all bronchi down to subsegmental level in all lobes of the lung.

Additional procedures during fibreoptic bronchoscopy if required
- Aspiration of secretions through the suction channel for microbiological or cytological examination
- Biopsy of tracheal or bronchial mucosa for diagnosis of suspected tumour or other conditions such as sarcoidosis (see Chapter 11)
- Transbronchial biopsy of diffuse or localised pulmonary opacities. The biopsy forceps are advanced through the wall of the bronchus under direct vision and aided by fluoroscopy, into the abnormal area of lung or into the opacity
- An abrasive sterile brush can be passed through the bronchoscope to collect cellular material and secretions from abnormal areas for cytological or microbiological examination. Special catheters are available to minimise contamination of material by upper respiratory tract organisms and are especially valuable in investigation of infection in the immune deficient host (see Chapter 20)
- Lavage of the bronchi and alveoli of a segment or lobe with saline for microbiological and cytological examination
- Transbronchial needle biopsy of sub-carinal lymph nodes for cytological evidence of carcinoma
- Bronchography for diagnosis of bronchiectasis or less often for identification of peripheral bronchial carcinomas or bronchial stenosis of any cause (see Chapter 6).

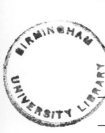

RIGID BRONCHOSCOPY

Although the development of fibreoptic bronchoscopy has greatly reduced the need for rigid bronchoscopy, there are several clinical situations in which we believe rigid bronchoscopy with general anaesthesia to be superior.

1. Children
2. Removal of foreign bodies (see Chapter 24)
3. Emergency treatment of large haemoptysis (see Chapter 3)
4. Suspected tumours of the trachea or carina. Small amounts of bleeding after biopsy can obstruct breathing and an adequate airway is easier to ensure with the rigid bronchoscope
5. Suspicion of a lesion which might bleed profusely on biopsy
6. Many surgeons prefer personally to assess operability of bronchial carcinoma by rigid bronchoscopy especially if the site of the tumour may lead to a decision between lobectomy or pneumonectomy.

11. BIOPSY OF THE LUNG

Biopsy of the lung is a highly specialised procedure, the technical details of which will not be described here. The clinical usefulness of lung biopsy and the choice of technique are discussed in several other chapters of this book. The main methods available are:
— Open 'surgical' biopsy
— Transbronchial biopsy through the fibreoptic bronchoscope
— Percutaneous biopsy
Fine needle or cutting needle
High speed trephine ('drill')

Surgical biopsy

This is most commonly used for diagnosis of diffuse lung diseases as it provides a specimen of sufficient size for detailed histological, microbiological and other examinations and lessens the problems of sampling from what may be patchy disease. Open biopsy is occasionally required for more localised disease if, for example, an uncontaminated specimen is required and percutaneous biopsy techniques are inappropriate. Many consider that open biopsy is, paradoxically, the least dangerous technique in severely ill patients with a bleeding tendency because of better control of haemorrhage. It is of course essential to discuss the clinical problem in detail with the thoracic surgeon and, in a very sick patient, with the anaesthetist. In diffuse disease it is advisable to request that a lobe other than the lingula is biopsied as the pathological appearances in the lingula are said to differ from the rest of the lung. It is essential to inform the surgeon if all or part of the specimen must be specially handled or placed in special media for microbiology or electron microscopy or immunofluorescence studies

Transbronchial biopsy

This is performed at fibreoptic bronchoscopy and the technique and indications are described in Chapter 10

Percutaneous biopsy techniques

Percutaneous biopsy techniques are rapid, are carried out with local anaesthesia and should be painless. The choice between them should be based not only on the clinical problem but also on the experience, expertise and previous success of those who are to carry out the procedure.

— *Needle biopsy.* A special 20 or 21 gauge needle is introduced under fluoroscopic guidance into the radiologically abnormal area. Samples may be obtained by aspiration or by the use of an inner screw stylet. Although ideally suited to obtaining a specimen for cytological examination small samples of tissue for histological examination can be obtained with the screw stylet. Pneumothorax occurs in 10–20% of patients but is usually small. This technique is mainly of value in biopsy of localised lesions but can be used to discover the causative organism in pneumonia.

The 'Trucut' or similar cutting needle can also be used to biopsy the lung in diffuse or localised disease. It is significantly larger than the above needle and carries a greater risk of pneumothorax and haemorrhage. Its main use is for biopsy of pleural masses but on occasion we have found it of value for biopsy of lung masses when it is necessary to obtain histological rather than cytological samples as, for example, if lymphoma or granuloma is suspected rather than carcinoma.

— *High speed trephine biopsy* ('*drill*' *biopsy*). A core of superficial lung tissue can be obtained by introducing a trephine rotated at high speed by an air drill. The specimen is usually of sufficient size to allow both histological and microbiological examination. The technique is most appropriate for diffuse lung disease as the needle cannot be guided radiographically, but it has been used for biopsy of the pleura. Approximately 25% of patients develop a pneumothorax. A small haemoptysis is not uncommon and life threatening or fatal haemotysis is probably more common than with other percutaneous techniques.

12. BIOPSY OF THE PLEURA

Indications

Pleural biopsy should be performed whenever a diagnostic aspiration is carried out in a patient with pleural effusion of unknown cause unless the fluid is purulent.

Pleural biopsy equipment

Abram's needle
The Abram's needle consists of three parts; (i) an inner stylet which is of little use during the procedure; (ii) a cylinder with a sharp end distally and a Luer-lock fitting proximally; and (iii) an outer tube with a pointed end and a window near the distal end. The open ended cylinder fits onto the outer tube by a spiral thread and biopsy is obtained by tightening this thread. This moves the inner cylinder with the sharp end across the open window of the outer tube and cuts off tissue in the window which falls into the lumen of the needle.

Trucut needle
This cutting needle is used to biopsy tissue from many sites of the body. Pleural fluid cannot be aspirated through the Trucut needle but the needle is very suitable for biopsy of thickened pleura when fluid is not present.

Technique of pleural biopsy (Abram's needle)

1. Explain the procedure to the patient and reassure him
2. Select the site for insertion of the biopsy needle and mark it in ink
3. Position the patient so that he is comfortable and so that you have good access to the site of insertion. The best position is usually sitting forwards with the arms resting on pillows
4. Sterilise the area around the insertion site with antiseptic e.g. iodine. Cover the patient's trousers or pyjamas with sterile drapes

5. Inject 1 or 2% lignocaine as local anaesthetic subcutaneously and then deeper through the chest wall. The anaesthetic should be given right down to the pleura and at this level intermittent aspiration through the needle will confirm whether the pleural cavity has been entered. If fluid is obtained then it is safe to proceed to biopsy the pleura
6. With a sharp scalpel cut through the skin and intercostal muscle
7. The biopsy needle is inserted through this track with a twisting motion. The neurovascular bundle runs near the lower edge of each rib and the biopsy needle must be inserted well away from this, just above a lower rib
8. When the pleural cavity has been entered fluid should be aspirated through the Abram's biopsy needle into a syringe and samples sent for examination (see Chapter 27). After this the pleural biopsy should be obtained. With the Abram's needle the conventional method is to withdraw the needle with the window open and facing in any direction *except upwards towards the neurovascular bundle*, until a resistance is felt which is interpreted as catching the pleura in the window. Rotation of the inner needle cuts off a piece of pleura which can then be drawn into the syringe with a small amount of pleural fluid. The procedure can be repeated without the need to remove the needle from the chest and at least three pleural biopsies are taken
9. If further aspiration of pleural fluid is required this can be drawn off through the biopsy needle as described in Chapter 27
10. When the needle is withdrawn the incision should be cleaned and either sprayed with a plastic spray or covered with Collodion and a dressing for 24 hours
11. Arrange chest X-ray to see whether a pneumothorax has been induced and to see how much fluid remains after aspiration.

13. TRANSTRACHEAL ASPIRATION

Transtracheal aspiration may be of value when tracheal or bronchial secretions, uncontaminated by oropharyngeal secretions, are required for analysis, (usually microbiological) as in:

— Immunosuppressed patients with pneumonia who can produce no sputum or whose sputum may be contaminated from the mouth or upper respiratory tract
— Patients with severe pneumonia when sputum has not yielded an organism and choice of treatment depends on obtaining a microbiological diagnosis
— Patients with pneumonia in whom infection is suspected with anaerobic bacteria or other unusual upper respiratory organisms which cannot be detected in sputum.

Transtracheal aspiration is not of value:

— When a proximal bronchial obstruction is suspected. Bronchoscopy is then preferable to confirm the obstruction and obtain a biopsy
— When lung tissue is required. Some opportunist infections such as pneumocystis may be more certainly diagnosed by examination of lung tissue and either bronchoscopy or percutaneous or open lung biopsy are then required (see Chapter 11).

Transtracheal aspiration should not be attempted:

— If there is a goitre overlying the cricothyroid membrane
— If there is any coagulation defect unless this can be corrected before the procedure. Thrombocytopenia is not a contraindication if a platelet transfusion can be given just before and during the transtracheal aspiration.

Technique

Like all technical procedures it is wise to seek tuition, or at least advice, before first embarking on this investigation.

1. It is essential to fully explain the procedure to the patient and give reassurance
2. Check all equipment
   a. A sharp scalpel blade (number 11)

   b. A cannula (e.g. 8 inch CVP line)
   c. 2, 10 and 20 ml syringes
   d. 10 ml vial of normal saline for injection
3. Position the patient carefully. Two pillows are placed under the shoulders and one under the head so that the neck is hyper-extended yet comfortable
4. Check the anatomical landmarks. Feel for the thyroid cartilage which is separated from the cricoid cartilage by the crico-thyroid membrane
5. Scrupulous sterile technique is essential. Sterilise a wide area of skin with iodine
6. Inject a small amount of lignocaine, 1% or 2%, subcutaneously over the cricothyroid membrane. Insert the needle through the crico-thyroid membrane into the trachea. Air can then be aspirated back into the syringe. Next, inject a small amount of lignocaine into the trachea. Warn the patient that he will cough but try to remove the needle before he does
7. With the scalpel blade make a small but fairly deep incision over the centre of the crico-thyroid membrane. Carefully insert the cannula through the crico-thyroid membrane taking care to penetrate in the mid line at right angles to the patient and pointing slightly towards his feet. Ask the patient not to cough, swallow or speak at this stage if possible. Thread the plastic inner cannula into the trachea through the trocar which is then withdrawn outside the neck and the guard attached to it
8. Suck secretions from the trachea into a 20 ml syringe. Usually very little material can be aspirated unless a small amount of normal saline is instilled into the trachea. Inject 1–2 ml at a time then ask the patient to take a few deep breaths followed by a couple of coughs while you apply suction with the syringe
9. Detach the syringe from the cannula and eject the material into a sterile container
10. Specimens should be sent for aerobic culture and sensitivity and, if indicated, for special stains and/or cultures for tuberculosis, pneumocystis or other organisms. Specimens for anaerobic culture should be sent in a syringe from which all the air has been expelled and which has an airtight cap
11. When adequate samples have been obtained withdraw the cannula steadily from the trachea. Seal the hole in the crico-thyroid membrane with collodion and apply a small adhesive dressing. The patient must not eat or drink for 2 hours after the procedure, and should be told to place his index finger over the adhesive dressing whenever he wishes to cough for the rest of the day

12. Careful observation is necessary for several hours after the aspiration to detect bleeding into the neck tracheal obstruction causing noisy or difficult breathing or an air leak.

Complications

— Haematoma can usually be avoided if any coagulation or platelet defect is corrected before aspiration is attempted and if pressure is applied to the crico-thyroid membrane immediately after the procedure and during coughing

— Surgical emphysema. Patients should be warned that this might occur but it should not do so if a finger is placed over the dressing whenever the patient coughs after the procedure. Surgical emphysema is of little clinical importance unless it is very extensive, in which case administration of high concentrations of oxygen and attempts to suppress cough may help

— Infection in the soft tissues of the neck is extremely rare

— Inhalation of material into the tracheo-bronchial tree may occur if the patient eats or drinks before the effects of the lignocaine have worn off.

14. SKIN TESTS FOR ATOPY

Skin tests offer a means of identifying individuals who produce excessive specific IgE to common allergens i.e. who are atopic.

Technique

1. The patient must be instructed not to take any antihistamine-containing drug for 24 hours before testing.
2. Choice of antigens. Most atopic patients in the UK react to one or more of the following antigens:
   — House dust mite
   — Grass pollen
   — Cat (or dog) hair
   — Aspergillus fumigatus
   If the purpose of testing is to identify atopic subjects there is little need to test other antigens
3. Put a drop of each antigen on the skin of the forearm, and also drops of diluent (control) and dilute histamine solution. Mark the skin by each drop for identification
4. Using the point of a different intravenous needle for each drop 'lift' the skin under each without drawing blood
5. Wait 15–20 minutes then measure the diameter of each weal.

Interpretation

A weal 3 mm larger than the control is regarded as positive. It is best however to record the results as measured diameter of each weal. Erythema should be ignored. If a weal results from the control innoculation the test is difficult to interpret unless antigen solutions produce markedly larger responses. If no reaction is produced from the histamine inoculation, question the patient about antihistamine medication as this suppresses skin reactions.

Delayed reactions may develop 4–8 hours after skin testing, usually having been preceded by an immediate reaction soon after inoculation. Delayed reactions are less well defined than immediate reactions and usually do not irritate or itch. Therefore unless specifically sought they may be overlooked.

The uses of skin testing

— Skin testing is a reliable method of *identifying atopic subjects*. There is often little relationship between positive skin reactions and the clinical response of a patient's asthma or rhinitis to exposure to individual allergens, and individual reactions are little guide to the cause of symptoms or to their treatment.

— Demonstration of an immediate, with or without a delayed, response to aspergillus fumigatus aids *diagnosis of allergic broncho-pulmonary aspergillosis* (see Chapter 30)

— The diagnosis of *some forms of occupational asthma* may be supported by a positive skin test (for example against complex platinum salts in workers with platinum asthma).

— Now that immunotherapy is less commonly used, this reason for performing detailed skin testing no longer holds

15. TUBERCULIN SKIN TEST

The development of induration 2–4 days after the intradermal injection of tuberculin indicates presents or previous infection with *M. tuberculosis*, related mycobacteria or BCB. Several methods are available:

The Mantoux test

0.1 ml of a purified protein derivative of tuberculin (PPD) is injected intradermally into the volar surface of the forearm (to raise a bleb). This volume of the 1 in 1000 PPD preparation available in the UK contains 10 tuberculin units (10 TU). This is the strength most commonly used in practice but dilutions of 1 TU (1 in 10 000 tuberculin) or 100 TU (1 in 100 tuberculin) are available for special purposes. Old tuberculin is no longer used.

The Mantoux test requires some skill but is the standard against which other methods have been compared. There is however much variation in the preparations of tuberculin available in different countries, and dilute solutions are unstable.

The reaction is read at 48–72 hours by measuring the diameter of induration. Any erythema is ignored. The result should be recorded as the measured diameter of the reaction rather than 'positive' or 'negative'. Induration of 5 mm or greater diameter to 10 TU is considered 'positive' in the UK but WHO recommends that a reaction of 10 mm to 5 TU be considered 'positive'.

The Heaf multiple puncture test

A drop of a more concentrated PPD preparation is placed on the skin of the forearm and intradermal inoculation is obtained by releasing a spring loaded 'gun' which carries 6 short steel needles which penetrate the skin to a depth of 2 mm (this can be adjusted to 1 mm for use in babies or younger children).

The Heaf test is easy to perform and does not face children with the threat of a visible needle. It is easier and quicker than the Mantoux test to perform on large numbers. The reaction is read between 72 hours and 4 days.

The results are graded. The test is negative grade 0 if there is no palpable induration. Grade 1 (4 or more palpable papules), grade 2 (papules form a ring of induration), grade 3 (the centre of the ring of induration is filled), grade 4 (vesiculation or induration of more than 10 mm diameter). Grade 3 and 4 are usually considered 'positive' but it is preferable to record the grade of reaction on the records rather than merely 'positive' or 'negative'.

Tine test

Four sharp needles (tines) are coated with sterile dried tuberculin and mounted in a small disposable plastic holder. The tines are pressed on the skin of the volar surface of the forearm to produce four puncture sites.

The tine test has suffered from problems of irregular coating of tuberculin on the tines with resulting false negative reactions, and we do not recommend its use.

Imotest

The imotest has recently been introduced as a convenient disposable unit. The tuberculin liquid is squeezed from a small plastic tube onto the points which are pressed into the skin. Palpable induration greater than 3 mm diameter is regarded as 'positive', equivalent to 5 TU PPD in the Mantoux test. Induration between 1 and 3 mm diameter is 'doubtfully positive' and smaller or absent reactions are 'negative'.

Significance of a positive tuberculin test

— Present or previous infection with *M. tuberculosis*
— Present or previous infection with other mycobacteria
— Previous BCG immunisation.

Significance of small tuberculin reactions

— Waning sensitivity many years after infection or BCG immunisation
— A very recent primary infection (within previous 6 weeks)
— Present or previous infection with mycobacteria other than *M. tuberculosis*
— Test incorrectly performed or read, or tuberculin of declining potency.

Significance of a negative tuberculin test

— No previous infection with *M. tuberculosis*
— The test is negative in 3–10% of patients with active tuberculosis, especially in the very ill, elderly or those with overwhelming miliary or meningeal tuberculosis.
— Transient suppression of a previously positive reaction may occur during virus infections such as measles or influenza
— Depression of previously positive reactions in patients who develop sarcoidosis, Hodgkin's disease, other lymphomas or leukaemia or who have widespread malignancy
— Depression of previously positive reactions during treatment with systemic corticosteroids at high dosage
— Test incorrectly performed or inadequate materials used.

Clinical usefulness of the tuberculin test

The tuberculin test is of limited value in investigation of an individual suspected of having tuberculosis as, although a strongly positive reaction may increase suspicion, a negative reaction does not exclude the disease. The test is obviously of greater diagnostic value in young people who have not received BCG than in older people who may either have received BCG or may have previous tuberculosis, now healed, which is unrelated to the condition now under investigation. Tuberculin testing is of greater value in the investigation of tuberculosis contacts, particularly children, who have not received BCG. It is also widely applied in the UK to assess the need for BCG immunisation of children and, indirectly, as a measure of the prevalence of tuberculosis in the community.

Section 3
SOME COMMON PROBLEMS

16. RESPIRATORY FAILURE

Respiratory failure may result from:
— Lung disorders, by causing disturbance of either ventilation or of blood flow *or*
— disorders of the chest wall or diaphragm or neuromuscular disease.

Respiratory failure may develop rapidly or slowly and may be transient or persistent. It is present when failure of gas exchange results in lowered arterial tension of oxygen (Pao_2 lower than 8.0 KPa) either alone or together with elevated tension of carbon dioxide ($Paco_2$ over 6.5 KPa).

Respiratory failure is suspected from the clinical setting and clinical examination and is confirmed by measuring arterial blood gas tensions (see Chapter 8).

Consider respiratory failure when a patient:
— is breathless at rest
— has central cyanosis
— has a raised respiratory rate
— is drowsy, confused or unconscious.

Measure arterial blood gases in all such patients.

Four types of respiratory failure can be recognised:
1. Acute hypoxia without hypercapnia
2. Chronic hypoxia without hypercapnia
3. Acute hypoxia with hypercapnia
4. Chronic hypoxia with hypercapnia.

Hypoxia is therefore invariable in respiratory failure and may or may not be accompanied by hypercapnia.

Because of the shape of the oxygen dissociation curve falls of Pao_2 to above 8.0 KPa have little effect on oxygen saturation and little effect on tissue oxygen supplies. Below this level however further falls of Pao_2 results in a rapid fall of oxygen saturation.

ACUTE HYPOXIC RESPIRATORY FAILURE
(with normal or low $Paco_2$)

Commonly occurs in patients with:
— Acute asthma
— Pneumonia
— Pulmonary embolism
— Pulmonary oedema (of cardiac or non-cardiac cause)
— Pneumothorax

These disorders typically have an abrupt onset, often in patients
with previously normal lungs. In addition to the effects of the causative
illness, hypoxia itself leads to increased ventilation which often lowers
$Paco_2$. A sudden fall of Pao_2 to levels below about 7 KPa causes confusion
or even loss of consciousness.

Management

1. Treat the underlying condition
2. Give oxygen. All patients with severe acute hypoxia require
   oxygen. With the exception of certain patients (see caution
   below), it is safe to give oxygen at high concentration through
   any form of mask. A high concentration venturi mask has the
   advantage of delivering a constant concentration of oxygen,
   and knowledge of the concentration of inspired oxygen
   enables approximate calculations about gas exchange to be
   made (see below). We use a 40% or 60% venturi mask but,
   as many of these patients are hyperventilating, oxygen
   delivery is often below these values (see Chapter 40).
   Caution: When giving oxygen to a patient with previous
   chronic obstructive lung disease (such as chronic bronchitis or
   emphysema) or with severe chest wall or neuromuscular
   disease, start treatment with low concentrations of oxygen
   (e.g. 24%). It is essential to measure arterial blood gases
   soon afterwards to identify any rise of CO_2 tension
3. Repeat measurement of blood gases 30 minutes after starting
   oxygen therapy:
   a. to ensure that sufficient oxygen is being given to raise
      arterial Pao_2 to safe levels (over 7 KPa)
   b. to identify any developing hypercapnia.
      If arterial Pao_2 fails to rise sufficiently during oxygen
   therapy this may be due to what is, in effect, a right to left
   shunt in the lungs as underventilated lung continues to be
   perfused by pulmonary arterial blood. The magnitude of such
   a shunt can be calculated approximately as a guide to further
   treatment:

Thus if 40% oxygen is administered:
— with no shunt Pao_2 should be 32 KPa
— with a 10% shunt Pao_2 will be 18 KPa
— with a 25% shunt Pao_2 will be 10 KPa
If a large shunt is present increasing concentrations of inspired oxygen can have little effect on arterial Pao_2

4. Most patients with acute hypoxic respiratory failure recover with treatment of the underlying disease and with oxygen therapy but *consider assisted ventilation* if:
   a. Pao_2 cannot be raised to a safe level (over 7 KPa) with oxygen therapy at hight concentrations (e.g. 60%)
   b. A safe level of Pao_2 is achieved but only at the expense of unacceptable respiratory effort with tachypnoea, distress or exhaustion. If such a situation is ignored further deterioration may lead to cardiorespiratory arrest
   c. Hypercapnia develops which cannot be reversed by energetic attempts to remove secretions (if present) or by treatment of the underlying disease.

CHRONIC HYPOXIC RESPIRATORY FAILURE (with normal or low $Paco_2$)

Chronic hypoxic respiratory failure may develop as a result of any chronic lung disease which alters the distribution of ventilation and/or perfusion.

A slowly developing fall of Pao_2 usually causes little or no loss of mental activity or confusion, such as occurs in acute hypoxia. Similarly there may be no breathlessness at rest. Evidence may be found of the physiological responses to chronic hypoxia such as pulmonary hypertension or secondary polycythaemia.

Consider chronic hypoxic respiratory failure in patients with:
— Chronic obstructive bronchitis
— Emphysema
— Widespread pulmonary fibrosis
— Chronic chest wall or neuromuscular disease
— Chronic thrombo-embolism
when they complain of:
— Ankle oedema
— Awakening at night or repeated nightmares.
The only constant sign is central cyanosis.

Investigations

— Arterial blood gases (see Chapter 8)
— Blood count. Haemoglobin and packed cell volume (PCV) are often raised (secondary polycythaemia) but beware 'spurious polycythaemia' due to low plasma volume if the patient has received diuretics
— ECG may show P pulmonale, right axis deviation, right bundle branch block or signs of right ventricular hypertrophy
— Chest X-ray to:
  — assist diagnosis of the underlying cause
  — assess cardiac enlargement
  — assess enlargement of proximal pulmonary arteries.

Management

1. Treat the underlying disease
2. Oxygen. Unlike the patient with acute hypoxia, the patient with chronic hypoxic respiratory failure is often not in immediate need of oxygen.
   Oxygen is needed:
   a. if there is a further acute fall of Pao_2
   b. if it is to be given as a long-term treatment. (see Chapter 38)
      Patients with severe chronic airflow obstruction or chest wall or neurological disorders are at risk of developing hypercapnea during acute respiratory illnesses and caution is needed in prescribing oxygen. The risk of hypercapnia developing in patients with chronic hypoxia from other causes is much less but it is usually advisable to start oxygen therapy with low inspired concentrations (e.g. 24% or 2 litres per minute)
3. Long-term oxygen therapy (see Chapter 39)
4. Repeat arterial blood gas measurements to assess the improvement of Pao_2 and to detect any hypercapnia
5. Venesection (or erythrophoresis). Reduction of the haematocrit in patients with severe secondary polycythaemia may improve symptoms but seems to be effective only if Hb is greater than 18 g/dl and PCV greater than 60%. It is advisable to confirm that these high values are due to polycythaemia rather than a low plasma volume by measuring red cell mass using a radioisotopic method.
   For venesection, using a standard blood donor collection set, blood is collected from an antecubital vein into the collecting bag. Simultaneously an equal volume of Dextran 40 is infused into a vein in the other arm to prevent a sudden reduction of circulating blood volume. It is unwise to remove more than 1 litre of blood in 24 hours.

Erythrophoresis is a newer technique requiring expensive equipment which seperates red cells from blood, returning plasma to the patient.

Both techniques are intended to reduce PCV to about 45% and may be repeated at intervals if need be. Repeated removal of red cells may lead to iron deficiency and such patients require oral iron supplements.

Increasing use of long-term oxygen therapy, which also brings about a reduction of secondary polycythaemia, may reduce the need for venesection

6. Diuretics. Peripheral oedema in chronic hypoxic patients may improve with reduction of hypoxaemia but diuretics are often required. Loop diuretics such as frusemide or bumetanide together with potassium-sparing agents such as spironolactone, triamterine or amiloride are preferred. As well as reducing discomfort and weight of the legs diuretics probably have beneficial haemodynamic effects.

ACUTE HYPOXIA WITH HYPERCAPNIA (Pa_{O_2} less than 8 KPa, Pa_{CO_2} greater than 6.5 KPa)

Elevation of Pa_{CO_2} implies inadequate ventilation such that CO_2 production exceeds loss of CO_2 from the lungs. High alveolar CO_2 tension is inevitably accompanied by low O_2 tension so that hypoxia is invariable in a patient with raised Pa_{CO_2} who is breathing air.

Acute hypoxia with hypercapnia may result from:

Failure of respiratory drive:
— Respiratory depressant drugs (e.g. diazepam, opiates or alcohol)
— Acute neurological disease (e.g. brain stem damage from stroke or trauma).

Failure of transmission of respiratory drive (see Chapter 28):
— Disorders of nerves or neuromuscular transmission (e.g. acute polyneurites of Guillain-Barré, paraplegia, poliomyelitis, myasthenia gravis or curarisation)
— Disorders of muscle affecting respiratory muscles (e.g. acute polymyositis)
— Disorders of chest wall may be acute (trauma) but are more often chronic (scoliosis, thoracoplasty, gross obesity, extensive pleural fibrosis) in which case acute respiratory failure of this type may develop during intercurrent respiratory illness.

Failure of the lungs to respond to respiratory drive.
— Severe airflow obstruction (e.g. acute asthma, exacerbation of chronic bronchitis, laryngeal or tracheal obstruction)

— Stiff lungs (e.g. severe pneumonia, pulmonary oedema)
— Large pneumothorax or pleural effusion can mechanically impede ventilation despite normal or increased neurological respiratory drive and normal transmission of drive.

Note: Hypoxia with hypercapnia frequently occurs in the absence of lung disease (as in cases 1 & 2 above) the commonest causes of this type of respiratory failure in hospital practice probably being acute stroke or self-administered drug overdosage.

Suspect acute hypoxia with hypercapnia when a patient with one of the above conditions develops:
— Drowsiness or confusion, often with headache
— Tachycardia
— Tremor
— Peripheral vasodilation (flushed appearance, warm hands and feet and bounding pulse).

The clinical features depend upon the level and rate of increase of $Paco_2$ and upon the underlying disorder.

Arterial blood gas analysis not only confirms the presence of hypoxia and hypercapnia but may provide a clue to the acuteness of the rise of $Paco_2$. Renal retention of bicarbonate takes time to occur so that a normal level of bicarbonate (or base excess) in a patient with high $Paco_2$ suggests recent respiratory failure (unless there is some other cause of metabolic acidosis such as renal failure, diabetic ketoacidosis or very severe hypoxia, or unless renal tubular function is impaired).

Management

1. Acute respiratory failure of this type is a medical emergency requiring immediate treatment
2. Treat the underlying condition if possible
3. No recognised or possible respiratory depressant drug must be given to any patient with raised $Paco_2$ unless the risk of doing so is accepted and facilities are available to support ventilation. This warning applies to all analgesic, sedative, hypnotic or antidepressant agents
4. Oxygen therapy. If the rise of $Paco_2$ has been recent there is relatively little risk of increasing hypoventilation by giving oxygen. However, it is not possible to be certain that administration of oxygen will not reduce a hypoxic drive to ventilation and, in addition, such patients are at risk of a further fall of ventilation if the underlying condition worsens. It is wise therefore to start with 24% oxygen with the purpose of achieving a safe but still below normal Pao_2 (see

Chapter 29). This must be followed by repeated measurements of arterial gas tensions until a safe level of Pao_2 has been achieved (Pao_2 over 7 KPa) and $Paco_2$ is stable or preferably falling. Very careful observation is required and any increase in drowsiness or any clinical deterioration should lead to further measurement of arterial blood gases

5. Removal of secretions: all patients with chronic bronchitis and those with sputum from any other cause must be encouraged to cough. Such patients, although often drowsy and unwell, must be persuaded to cough at least every 2 hours and preferably more often.

   Emergency bronchoscopy is very occasionally required to remove secretions if airflow obstruction is thought to be mainly due to retention of sputum, or if there is lobar collapse due to retained secretions

6. Bronchodilator drugs (see Chapter 30) should be given, most conveniently by nebulisation, if there is airflow obstruction (chronic bronchitis, emphysema, asthma)

7. Stimulant drugs are clearly of little value for patients whose respiratory failure is due to failure of respiratory drive or failure of transmission of respiratory drive. Likewise they are ineffective, and possibly dangerous, in patients with stiff lungs or asthma. In treatment of respiratory failure complicating chronic bronchitis, stimulant drugs have been advocated for two purposes:

   Cerebral stimulants (such as nikethamide 5–10 ml of 25% solution slowly I.V.) may temporarily waken the drowsy patient who can then be encouraged to cough. This can be achieved only once or twice, is transient, and carries the small risk of causing convulsions.

   Respiratory stimulant drugs (such as doxapram hydrochloride 0.5–4.0 mg per minute) are intended to increase or maintain ventilation for a short time, at most 24 hours. Their use may allow oxygen therapy to be given at a concentration which, without stimulant, caused a rise of $Paco_2$.

   The role of doxapram is not generally agreed but it may 'buy time' while other energetic treatment is given in an attempt to avoid the need for assisted ventilation

8. Assisted ventilation must be considered if safe levels of Pao_2 and $Paco_2$ cannot be obtained with other treatments.
   a. In conditions other than chronic bronchitis, assisted ventilation is required if rapid improvement of severe hypoxia and hypercapnia cannot be obtained and if recovery is possible. If not ventilated such patients are at risk of sudden death especially during sleep.

External negative pressure ventilation (with a tank
respiratory or a cuirass) may be appropriate for patients
with chest wall or neuromuscular disorder if they:
(i) are conscious
(ii) have a functioning larynx to present aspiration.
b. For treatment of an exacerbation of chronic bronchitis the
decision whether, and when, to advise assisted ventilation
is difficult because most such patients will have been
severly disabled by their disease for a long time before the
present episode and because episodes of respiratory failure
may occur repeatedly.

Before advising assisted ventilation consider:
— Are there any potentially treatable factors (such as recent
infection, respiratory depressant drugs, rib fracture etc)? If
not assisted ventilation will not lead to recovery
— Was the quality of the life before this setback such as to
justify prolonging life by assisted ventilation? This decision
can be made only by someone who knew the patient
before the present episode or after discussion with such a
person
— Are there any special risks of assisted ventilation for this
patient?
— Was lung function so poor before this episode that it may
be impossible to discontinue assisted ventilation after this
acute episode?
— What was the outcome of any previous episodes of
respiratory failure?
If assisted ventilation is required then the aid of an
experienced anaesthetist is needed for endotracheal
intubation and subsequent care. Details of management
during assisted ventilation are outside the scope of this
book.

CHRONIC HYPOXIA WITH HYPERCAPNIA

Chronic hypoxia with hypercapnia may develop in patients with:
— Severe chronic bronchitis and emphysema
— Chest wall abnormalities including gross obesity, scoliosis,
muscle weakness (see Chapter 28)
— Central hypoventilation.
Such patients often tolerate raised Pa_{CO_2} and low Pa_{O_2} without marked
impairment of mental function. In addition to symptoms of chronic
hypoxia headache, particularly in the morning, is a common symptom.

Management

1. Except in the case of obesity there is usually little improvement of the underlying disease possible by the stage of chronic respiratory failure but efforts should nevertheless be made to search for any treatable factors and deal with them appropriately

2. Oxygen therapy carries the risk of causing depression of ventilation if respiratory drive has been dependant on hypoxia. Correction of hypoxia will then cause a further rise of $Paco_2$ resulting in confusion, drowsiness or loss of consciousness. *Think carefully before prescribing oxygen to such patients*, for once $Paco_2$ has risen as a result of oxygen administration, it does not necessarily fall again if oxygen is withdrawn. Withdrawal of oxygen merely leaves the patient with a higher $Paco_2$ and hence a lower Pao_2 than before treatment was started.

   Oxygen is usually required:
   — for worsening of the underlying condition
   — during intercurrent illnesses which result in worsening of arterial gases
   — as a long-term treatment (usually contraindicated in the presence of raised $Paco_2$).

   a. It is essential to measure arterial blood gases before starting oxygen therapy
   b. Give not more than 24% oxygen (Venturi mask)
   c. Repeat blood gas analysis after 30 minutes and again after 1 to 2 hours, or sooner if the patient becomes drowsy. If there is obvious improvement of mental state further arterial samples may not be required
   d. A small rise of $Paco_2$ often occurs soon after starting oxygen but this is usually not accompanied by more than a small increase in acidosis (because of the buffering capacity of the blood). If no further rise occurs oxygen can be continuted at that concentration
   e. *Give oxygen continuously and not intermittently.* The rapid fall of Pao_2 whenever oxygen is withdrawn may be hazardous. Because of the need for continuous treatment nasal oxygen (1–2 l/min) is often preferred to a mask after the first few hours of treatment
   f. Oxygen concentration can be increased to 28% if a safe level of Pao_2 (over 7 KPa) is not achieved on 24% oxygen and if $Paco_2$ is stable
   g. Whenever the concentration of oxygen is increased arterial blood must be analysed within 1 hour to identify any further rise of $Paco_2$

3. Respiratory stimulant drugs (see p 73) may produce temporary improvement, either to enable oxygen therapy to be continued in the face of a rising arterial P_{CO_2}, or to 'buy time' for physiotherapy, antibiotics or bronchodilator therapy to take effect.

4. Assisted ventilation (see p 74). In the patient with chronic lung disease assisted ventilation is not appropriate for the treatment of chronic respiratory failure of this type, but may be life-saving during an acute episode in which arterial P_{CO_2} rises still further (see p 74). Tank or curaisse respirators may be appropriate for some patients with normal lungs (see Chapter 28) and may sometimes need to be continued indefinitely.

NOCTURNAL RESPIRATORY FAILURE

Nocturnal hypoventilation results in hypoxia and hypercapnia intermittently during sleep.

It may result from:

— Obstruction to breathing during sleep, usually in the upper airway
— Reduction of respiratory drive during sleep.

Suspect nocturnal hypoventilation in a patient with:

— Daytime somnolence or personality change (due to frequent arousal from sleep as a result of hypoxia)
— Early morning headaches
— Secondary polycythaemia or pulmonary hypertension without other cause
— Nocturnal cardiac dysrhythmias
— Loud snoring during sleep in association with any of the above.

Nocturnal hypoventilation may occur in patients with:

— Severe chronic bronchitis, asthma or cystic fibrosis
— Normal lungs with:
  — chest wall or neuromuscular disorders (see Chapter 28)
  — upper airways obstruction (obesity, enlarged adenoids)
  — central sleep apnoea of neurological cause

The diagnosis is confirmed by specialised techniques including continuous measurement of P_{aO_2} during sleep (ear oximeter or transcutaneous electrodes) which detect periods of hypoxia, ideally with parallel measurements of P_{aCO_2} and of respiratory movements (see Chapter 28).

17. PULMONARY HYPERTENSION

Pulmonary hypertension is less common than systemic hypertension but, unlike the latter, a cause is usually found.
Pulmonary artery pressure = (Cardiac output × pulmonary vascular resistance) + left atrial pressure.

Hence pulmonary hypertension can result from:

Increased cardiac output. Physiological increases of cardiac output which occur during exercise or pregnancy have little effect on pulmonary artery pressure. Pulmonary blood flow must increase to many times normal to significantly increase pulmonary artery pressure. This occurs in congenital shunts such as patent ductus arteriosus, and atrial or ventricular septal defects

Increased pulmonary vascular resistance which may be due to:
a. vasoconstriction – as occurs in hypoxia.
b. obstruction of arteries – pulmonary emboli
c. loss of vessels – emphysema, lung resection, severe scoliosis
d. hyperviscosity states – polycythaemia, myeloma
e. disease of pulmonary vessels – systemic sclerosis, widespread pulmonary vasculitis, or primary pulmonary hypertension.

Raised left atrial pressure resulting from:
a. left ventricular failure
b. mitral stenosis
c. left atrial myxoma

Hence in practice pulmonary hypertension is seen most often as a complication of a previously recognised respiratory or cardiac disorder but occasionally the dominant symptoms and signs are due to the pulmonary hypertension itself.

The symptoms, signs and X-ray appearances are those of the underlying disease with additional features due to pulmonary hypertension.

Diagnosis of pulmonary hypertension

Suspect pulmonary hypertension in a patient with some or all of the following symptoms or signs:

Symptoms
— Breathlessness on effort
— Fatigue
— Angina
— Syncope on effort
— Peripheral oedema
(plus of course, symptoms of the underlying disease).

Signs
— Small volume arterial pulse
— Right ventricular heave
— Prominent a wave in jugular venous pulse with or without raised pressure
— Loud pulmonary second sound.

There may in addition be a pulmonary systolic murmur, a pulmonary ejection click or signs of pulmonary and/or tricuspid incompetence.

Investigations

The following investigations may support the diagnosis of pulmonary hypertension:

Chest X-ray (in addition to features of any underlying disease) may show:
— Large main pulmonary artery and proximal arteries
— Reduction in size and number of vessels in periphery of lungs and sometimes an enlarged heart.

Electrocardiogram may show:
— Right axis deviation
— Right bundle branch block
— Tall P waves in right chest leads
— ST and T inversion in right chest leads.

Echocardiogram may show:
— Thick right ventricular wall
— Dilated right ventricular cavity
   N.B. The mitral valve and left atrium must be carefully examined.
   Pulmonary artery catheterisation is not necessary in all patients to confirm the presence of pulmonary hypertension. If characteristic changes of X-ray, ECG and echocardiogram are present in a patient who has a recognised cause of pulmonary hypertension, catheterisation is needed only if measurement of pulmonary artery pressure, cardiac output or pulmonary vascular resistance will influence or guide treatment or if some additional cause is suspected.

Diagnosis of the cause of pulmonary hypertension

Are any of the common causes known to be present?
- Severe chronic bronchitis and emphysema
- Known congenital heart disease
- Mitral stenosis
- Recurrent pulmonary embolism
- Severe scoliosis or other chest deformity
- Severe neuromuscular disorder
- Gross obesity.

If none of these are evident on clinical examination or from the history:
- Mitral stenosis should still be considered because of the occasional difficulty of diagnosis and the effectiveness of surgical treatment. In severe pulmonary hypertension no diastolic murmur may be heard and an opening snap may merge with the loud pulmonary second sound. Chest X-ray may show an enlarged left atrium, a calcified mitral valve or septal lines. An echocardiogram may confirm or exclude rheumatic mitral valve disease (or left atrial myxoma). Cardiac catheterisation may show a high wedge pressure but this may be unobtainable if there is severe pulmonary vascular narrowing in which case direct measurement of left atrial pressure may be required
- Enquire again about any episodes which, in retrospect, might have been due to pulmonary emboli e.g. recurrent syncope, pneumonias, unexplained pleurisy, haemoptyses
- Enquire carefully about any features to suggest nocturnal hypoventilation? (see Chapter 16) such as disturbed sleep, daytime somnolence, snoring, early morning headache
- Look specifically for any features of scleroderma or of the 'CREST' syndrome (Raynaud's phenomenon, calcinosis, sclerodactyly, telangiectasia)
- Ask about any travel to areas of endemic schistosomiasis
- Enquire whether the patient is orthopnoeic? This may suggest left ventricular failure or mitral stenosis or pulmonary veno-occlusive disease
- Enquire closely about the onset of symptoms in relation to pregnancy, venous thrombosis or surgical operation which may suggest thromboembolism
- Look for any features to suggest systemic lupus or generalised vasculitis

In the absence of any such clues the diagnosis usually rests between thromboembolic or primary pulmonary hypertension.

Further investigations

Arterial blood gases – hypoxia may result from severe pulmonary hypertension or may be the cause. Normal arterial oxygen tensions by day do not discount nocturnal hypoxia as a cause, for which measurement of Pao_2 during sleep is necessary (see Chapter 16)

Investigate to exclude hyperviscosity states

Lung function tests. Standard tests are often normal in the absence of underlying lung disease but carbon monoxide gas transfer may be low

Antinuclear factor, rheumatoid factor (and other tests for connective tissue disorders) should be measured

Isotope ventilation and perfusion scans may show abnormalities related to the underlying disease be it pulmonary or cardiac. Scans may help to distinguish between thromboembolic disease in which there may be multiple perfusion defects, and primary pulmonary hypertension, in which perfusion scans are normal

Cardiac catheterisation will confirm high pulmonary artery pressure and enable cardiac output to be measured. An intracardiac shunt can be recognised. A raised pulmonary wedge pressure suggests mitral stenosis, left atrial myxoma, left ventricular failure or pulmonary veno-occlusive disease (although this may not always cause a raised wedge pressure)

Pulmonary angiogram will demonstrate occlusion of large pulmonary arteries by embolism but it is very difficult to distinguish between widespread occlusion of small pulmonary artery branches by emboli or other causes of pulmonary hypertension. Pulmonary angiography carries an increased risk in the presence of severe pulmonary vascular obstruction and this risk must be weighed against the therapeutic usefulness of any information that might be obtained

Open lung biopsy is required for diagnosis of pulmonary veno-occlusive disease or possibly of widespread pulmonary vasculitis, but is rarely necessary otherwise. The operation carries a significant risk in a patient with severe pulmonary hypertension.

Management

In the commonest situation when pulmonary hypertension is secondary to chronic lung disease, treatment is aimed at the underlying disease in the hope that pulmonary hypertension will thereby improve. Long-term nocturnal oxygen therapy is discussed in Chapters 29 and 39.

1. For some underlying conditions specific treatment may be possible, for example:
   — surgical correction of congenital heart disease or of mitral valve disease
   — correction of hyperviscosity state
   — nocturnal ventilatory support for patients with scoliosis or neuromuscular disease
   — treatment of nocturnal hypoventilation
2. Anticoagulants have been advocated to prevent further episodes of embolism in thromboembolic pulmonary hypertension or possibly to prevent pulmonary artery thrombosis in pulmonary hypertension of other causes, but there is little evidence that this treatment is effective
3. Pulmonary vasodilator dugs may reduce pulmonary artery pressure but toxicity and adverse effects often limit their use and the results of oral treatment are disappointing. Hydrallazine, diazoxide, nifedipine and, more recently, intravenous prostacyclin have been used, mainly in treatment of primary pulmonary hypertension. This is a specialised form of treatment applicable to only a few patients with pulmonary hypertension. It requires careful initial assessment of the patient and repeated measurements of pulmonary artery pressure to assess the response
4. Heart failure is treated with diuretics
5. Heart-lung transplantation – this may be practicable for a very few young patients with no systemic disorder.

18. PNEUMONIA

Suspect pneumonia in an acute illness with:
- — Fever
- — Cough (with or without purulent sputum)
- — Breathlessness
- — Pleuritic pain

The clinical picture

This may differ in certain groups, for example:
- — Patients with chronic bronchitis may have a less acute illness with increased breathlessness and increased amounts of purulent sputum but little or no fever
- — The elderly may develop confusion or mental deterioration which overshadows respiratory symptoms
- — Patients in an intensive care unit, pneumonia may be suggested by an increased respiratory rate, fever, shadows on chest X-ray or fall of arterial Po_2
- — Among immunosuppressed patients, either a cough, fever or breathlessness alone should raise suspicion of pneumonia (see Chapter 20).

Physical examination

- — Fever (record temperature rectally or in the axilla if the patient is mouth breathing)
- — Central cyanosis
- — Herpes febrilis of the lips, especially in pneumococcal pneumonia
- — Breathing is rapid and may be shallow with grunting if there is pleuritic pain
- — Blood pressure may be low when pneumonia is associated with bacteraemia or severe hypoxaemia
- — The classical signs of consolidation are uncommon except in acute pneumococcal lobar pneumonia. Reduced movement, dullness to percussion and late inspiratory crackles may be the only abnormalities detected.

82

Chest X-ray (see also Chapter 37)

Both PA and lateral X-rays are required to be sure of detecting small
areas of consolidation, to distinguish consolidation from collapse and to
establish the site of shadowing in the lung.

Pneumonia usually causes an area of ill-defined shadowing within which
can often be seen areas of still aerated lung and/or air-filled bronchi ('air
bronchogram'). Occasionally pneumonia causes scattered ill-defined
opacities in several parts of the lung.

Lack of any loss of volume of the affected lobe (as shown by the
position of fissures, diaphragm and hila) and the presence of an air-
bronchogram make it unlikely that the bronchus is obstructed proximal to
the consolidation (by a tumour or foreign body).

Examine the costophrenic angles for pleural effusion.

Other investigations

White blood cell count and differential. A neutrophil
leucocytosis is common in primary bacterial pneumonia but
may not occur in pneumonia complicating chronic bronchitis,
surgical operations or old age. Neutropenia may occur in viral
pneumonia or with severe bacteraemic bacterial infection

Blood cultures are often positive especially in pneumococcal
pneumonia and are a more certain way of identifying the
organism that culture of potentially contaminated sputum

Sputum examination. Patients may be unable to produce
sputum in the early stages of pneumonia. Sputum
examination is of little value in management of pneumonia
complicating chronic bronchitis (see Chapter 29). Gram-
negative bacteria may be grown from sputum of patients who
have received wide spectrum antibiotics and this does not
necessarily reflect the cause of the pneumonia

Arterial blood gas analysis is not essential unless the patient
is very ill or has a history of severe chronic bronchitis or
other severe lung disease. Transient hypoxaemia is common
in pneumonia and reflects right to left shunting through
poorly ventilated lung. More severe hypoxaemia suggests
widespread pneumonia or severe underlying chronic lung
disease

Pa_{CO_2} is usually low in patients with pneumonia. A raised
level indicates overwhelming infection with failure of
respiratory drive or previous severe chronic bronchitis

Serological tests: Early diagnosis of legionella infection is now
available in some centres. Definite diagnosis of viral or
mycoplasma infection requires titration of acute and
convalescence sera. Detection of pneumococcal antigen in
sputum, urine or blood can speed the diagnosis of
pneumococcal pneumonia.

Clues to likely causes of pneumonia

Clinical clues

— Acute illness in a previously healthy person – *Strep. pneumoniae* (abrupt onset, herpes febrilis). *Mycoplasma pneumoniae* – antecedent malaise
— Acute illness during an influenza epidemic – *Strep. pneumoniae, Staph. pyogenes* (or rarely *Aspergillus fumigatus*)
— In a patient with chronic bronchitis – *Strep. pneumoniae, H. influenzae*
— After surgical operation, in old age or with general debility – upper respiratory organisms, anaerobic bacteria
— In an alcoholic – *Klebsiella*, tuberculosis, anaerobic bacteria
— With impaired immunity – see Chapter 20
— In an intensive care unit – Gram-negative bacteria
— Widespread pneumonia in a male homosexual or haemophiliac—consider pneumocystis complicating 'AIDS'.

Radiological clues to aetiology

— Lobar or segmental consolidation – *Strep. pneumoniae, Mycoplasma pneumoniae*
— Bilateral patchy consolidation – *Mycoplasma, Legionella, Psittacosis*
— Bilateral, lower zone – aspiration, 'hypostatic'
— Upper lobe or axilla with shrinkage or cavitation – aspiration (anaerobic bacteria), tuberculosis
— Cavitation – aspiration (anaerobes), *Staph. pyogenes, Klebsiella*, tuberculosis
— Diffuse 'haze' – *Pneumocystis*
— Nodules – fungi, septic emboli
— With pleural effusion – bacterial (especially pneumococcal)
— With calcification in lung – tuberculosis
— With adjacent periosteal reaction or rib destruction – actinomycosis.

MANAGEMENT

Not all patients with pneumonia are seriously ill. Depending on the patient's condition a decision must be reached whether to defer antibiotic therapy until microbiological information is available or to start treatment against the most likely infecting organism.

Oxygen

This should be given if the patient is cyanosed, confused or hypotensive. Arterial blood gases should be measured before starting oxygen therapy if there is a history of severe chronic bronchitis or emphysema. If Pa_{CO_2} is

normal or low, oxygen can be given by mask or nasal route at an initial
rate of 4 l/min or at a concentration of 35% but higher concentrations
may be needed and can be safely given. If Pa_{CO_2} is raised, see Chapter
16 for advice on oxygen therapy and possible ventilation. If the patient is
very sick, and safe arterial oxygen tensions (over 7 KPa) cannot be
obtained with high concentrations of inspired oxygen, assisted ventilation
may be necessary (see Chapter 16).

Hydration

Dehydration is common in patients with pneumonia. Fluids can often be
given by mouth but intravenous infusion is required if the patient is very
ill or is vomiting.

Relief of pleuritic pain

Non-steroidal anti-inflammatory agents such as indomethacin are
effective without suppressing respiration. Relief of pain is important to
facilitate effective coughing.

Cough

It is not wise to attempt to suppress cough with drugs. If the cough is
productive or if secretions can be heard 'bubbling' in the large airways
and if the patient cannot expectorate effectively then the help of a
physiotherapist should be sought (see Chapter 43).

Antibiotics

There are widely differing practices in the choice of antibiotics for
treatment of pneumonia and the range of available antibiotics increases
each year. We suggest some guidelines (written in 1985) but recognise
that local practice varies widely. There is rarely good evidence from
clinical trials by which to compare different regimens of treatment. The
doses suggested are for adults.

Before an organism has been demonstrated

Pneumonia acquired in the community by a previously healthy subject
— Patient in hospital but not severely ill. *Strep. pneumonia* is
the most likely cause but *M. pneumoniae, Legionella* or
Psitacosis must be considered. Oral or I.V. erythromycin
500 mg q.d.s.
— Patient severely ill. *Strep. pneumoniae* still most likely but
Staph. pyogenes, Legionella, H. influenzae or *psitticosis* are
important possibilities. I.V. erythromycin 1 g q.d.s.
plus I.V. cephalosporin (see footnote, p 86).

But during an epidemic of influenza there is a greater probability of *Staph. pyogenes*, therefore:

I.V. flucloxacillin 1.5 g q.d.s. plus I.V. gentamicin (according to renal function) plus I.V. erythromycin 1 g q.d.s.

Pneumonia acquired on a surgical ward
Consider Gram-negative bacteria, anaerobic organisms or *Staph. pyogenes*. I.V. cephalosporin (see footnote). If there is a real suspicion of aspiration or if there has been no improvement within 48 hours add I.V. metronidazole 500 mg t.d.s.

Pneumonia in a male homosexual or a haemophiliac
Consider pneumocystis complicating 'AIDS' and investigate further before treating.

Pneumonia acquired during artifical ventilation or on an intensive care unit
There are many possibilities including Gram-negative organisms such as *pseudomonas* or *Klebsiella* which may well be resistant to commonly used antibiotics. Rational treatment therefore requires laboratory examination of bronchial or tracheal secretions obtained by aspiration, through an endotracheal tube or tracheostomy, transtracheal aspiration through an 13) or bronchoscopy (see Chapter 10). Gram-negative bacteria are however commonly present in the trachea of sich patients without necessarily being the cause of their pneumonia. Isolation of organisms such as pseudomonas from bronchial or tracheal aspirates is not necessarily an indication for complex or potentially toxic regimes of antibiotic therapy.

Pneumonia complicating chronic bronchitis
— Patient not very ill from infection:
   oral ampicillin 500 mg q.d.s.
— Patient very ill from infection especially if recent antibiotics have been ineffective: consider *klebsiella, pseudomonas* or *legionella*: I.V. erythromycin 1 g q.d.s. plus I.V. cephalosporin (see footnote).

When laboratory evidence of infection has been obtained
— *Strep. pneumoniae*: If patient is improving on erythromycin or

---

FOOTNOTE
Injected cephalosporins
In the UK at the time of writing (1985) we consider the main use of cephalosporins in the treatment of pneumonia to be in the very sick patient, for whom we use cefotaxime; but other agents such as cefuroxime, ceftazidime, or ceftizoxime are available and equally effective.
   Suggested I.V. doses for adults with severe infections are:
   cefotaxime 2 g 3 times a day
   cefuroxime 1.5 g 8-hourly
   ceftazidime 1 g 8-hourly
   ceftizoxime 2 g 8-hourly
   (doses should reduced when renal function is impaired).
   This is a rapidly developing field and alternative cephalosporins are available in other countries and better compounds will doubtless be developed.

other antibiotic, continue. If not change to I.V. penicillin 1 mega unit q.d.s.
— *Staph. pyogenes*: I.V. flucloxacillin 1.5 g q.d.s. plus either I.V. gentamicin (according to renal function) or I.V. sodium fusidate 500 mg 8-hourly
— *Legionella*: I.V. erythromycin 1 g q.d.s.
— *H. influenzae*: I.V. cephalosporin
— *Psittacosis*: if patient is improving on erythromycin continue. If not change to I.V. tetracycline 500 mg q.d.s.

Interpretation of results of sputum culture

— If a patient is responding to the original antibiotic it is usually not necessary to change treatment because of the result of culture of sputum
— Gram-negative bacteria may be contaminants from the pharynx particularly if the patient has received previous antibiotics. Do not embark on a complex or toxic antibiotic treatment based on this information alone.

Assessment of response to treatment

The first indications of improvement are when the patient feels better and fever and respiratory and pulse rates fall. An increase in sputum volume is not an adverse sign if the patient is otherwise improving. Physical signs of consolidation may not improve for several days, and may persist for 1–2 weeks. Chest X-ray changes may not return to normal for 2 months or more.

Duration of treatment with antibiotics

There is little evidence upon which to base advice but our practice is:
— Acute pneumonia in previously healthy person 5–7 days
— Pneumonia complicating chronic bronchitis 7–10 days
— Aspiration or cavitating pneumonia 2–6 weeks.

Failure to respond to treatment

If the patient is still febrile and ill after 48 hours of antibiotic therapy, repeat the chest X-ray (PA and lateral):
1. Any pleural fluid, free or loculated? If so it is essential to aspirate fluid for microscopy and culture to confirm or exclude empyema (see Chapter 27). If more than a small amount of fluid is present it should be removed as completely as possible (see also management of empyema, Chapter 27)

    2. Any cavitation? This suggests abscess formation, infection
       with an unusual organism or an obstructed bronchus.
       Bronchoscopy is advisable to exclude the latter and obtain
       material for culture and microscopy
    3. Any extension of consolidation or any new shadows?

If so, review the diagnosis of pneumonia and consider conditions which
can be confused with pneumonia, such as:

    — Tuberculosis (see Chapter 21)
    — Pulmonary embolism (see Chapter 25)
    — Empyema (see Chapter 27)
    — Cavitating carcinoma (see Chapter 31)
    — Subphrenic abscess
    — Pulmonary eosinophilia (see Chapter 38)
    — Acute alveolitis (see Chapter 32)

If the diagnosis of pneumonia seems to be correct either change the
antibiotic or, much to be prefered, investigate the cause further by
bronchoscopy or transtracheal aspiration for culture of aspirate.

Unresolved or slowly resolving pneumonia

Abnormal shadowing may persist on chest X-ray for up to 2 months and
clearing is usually slower in the elderly and in those with pre-existing lung
disease. Residual scarring with loss of volume of the affected part of the
lung may follow pneumonia, particularly aspiration pneumonia and
particularly of an upper lobe.

    Persisting shadows may be pleural, either from pleural fibrosis or (of
great importance) from an empyema. The pleural nature should be
apparent if both PA and lateral X-rays are carefully examined and if the
possibility is considered. A persisting lobar or segmental shadow suggests
possible bronchial obstruction and bronchoscopy should be considered.
Persisting upper zone shadows may be due to tuberculosis – sputum
should be examined for mycobacteria.

Persisting or recurring fever after pneumonia

Consider the possibility of an empyema (see Chapter 27). PA and lateral
chest X-rays are necessary. Do not prescribe a further antibiotic until the
cause of the fever has been established.

19. LUNG ABSCESS

A lung abscess is a localised suppurating cavity within the lung.
Suspect a lung abscess when:

1. Purulent or offensive sputum, fever, sweating or weight loss follow a respiratory infection, surgical or dental operation or an episode of loss of consciousness
2. A cavitary opacity, or an air-fluid level within an area of consolidation, is seen on a chest X-ray.

COMMON CAUSES

Aspiration of infection from the upper respiratory tract particularly the nose, sinuses and pharynx (primary lung abscess). Such infections are usually with a mixture of anaerobic organisms with Gram-negative and Gram-positive bacteria. An initial pneumonia may develop into an abscess, or the abscess may be present when the patient is first seen. Abscess is more likely to occur when there is:

a. Ineffective cough (chest pain, debility)
b. Poor mucociliary clearance (chronic bronchitis)
c. Depressed consciousness (alcoholics, epilepsy, anaesthesia, drug overdose)
d. Non-functioning larynx (after topical local anaesthetics or in patients with bulbar palsy)
e. Upper respiratory infections (sinusitis) or dental infections
f. Gastro-oesophageal reflux or oesophageal obstruction (achalasia, peptic strictures, oesophageal carcinoma).

Specific pulmonary infections such as *Staph. pyogenes*, tuberculosis (tuberculous 'cavities' are merely abscesses), amoebiasis (sputum may resemble anchovy sauce), actinomycosis, fungal infections

Bronchial obstruction. Secretions distal to an obstruction (e.g. bronchial carcinoma, inhaled foreign body) are not cleared and may become infected

Septic emboli, usually staphylococcal, can cause multiple haematogenous lung abscesses as now often seen in 'main line' drug addicts
Secondarily infected pulmonary infarcts
Infected cysts (bronchogenic cysts, hydatid cysts, emphysematous bullae) or sequestrated segments.

OTHER CAUSES OF CAVITATING LESIONS ON CHEST X-RAY

— Cavitating pneumonia due to anaerobic organisms, *Klebsiella* or *staphylococcus pyogenes*. These infections cause lung destruction with multiple small abscesses
— Cavitating carcinoma, usually a squamous cell carcinoma
— Hiatus hernia. This may produce a fluid level seen behind the heart on the chest X-ray
— Empyema with broncho-pleural fistula. This may be difficult to distinguish from a peripheral lung abscess, as a fluid level is present on the X-ray and sputum is expectorated.
— Vasculitis e.g. Wegener's granuloma.

INVESTIGATION

Chest X-ray

(Both PA and lateral views are essential).
— Where is the abscess? Inhalation of infected material or foreign bodies occurs particularly into the lower lobes (especially the right), either in the basal or apical segments. Tuberculosis affects particularly the upper zones
— Are there multiple abscesses to suggest either necrotising pneumonia, tuberculosis, infarcts, or infected emboli?
— How thick is the cavity wall? Squamous carcinomas will often be thick walled, emphysematous bullae have thin hair-line edges on the chest X-ray
— Is the cavity in the centre of the lesion? It is often eccentric in cavitating carcinomas
— Is there loss of lobar volume or a mass to suggest a proximal bronchial obstruction from an inhaled foreign body or a bronchial carcinoma?
— Is there bone destruction to suggest carcinoma or, rarely infection, especially *actinomyces*?

Examination of sputum

Sputum should be examined for:
1. Anaerobic and microaerophilic bacteria (*Fusobacteria, Peptostreptococcus, Streptococcus milleri* etc). If anerobes are to be isolated sputum must be transferred immediately into an anaerobic atmosphere but even with these precautions it is difficult to isolate anaerobic bacteria from sputum
2. Tubercle bacilli. Large numbers of organisms are usually present in sputum from active cavitating tuberculosis
3. Aerobic bacteria (*Staphylococci, Klebsiella*)
4. Malignant cells.

When is further investigation necessary?

Bronchoscopy is strongly advised for all patients with a lung abscess unless tuberculosis has been diagnosed from sputum examination or a foreign body has been expectorated and the patient's condition and X-ray have improved. Rigid bronchoscopy is preferable if a foreign body might have been inhaled but otherwise a fibreoptic bronchoscopy is adequate. The bronchoscopist must be prepared to deal with the flow of pus which may be released from an abscess during the examination
Transbronchial aspiration or percutaneous needle aspiration of the abscess may be valuable if microbiological investigation of sputum is unhelpful and if identification of the organism is considered necessary as a guide to treatment. However it is usual to give a trial of antibiotics first.

TREATMENT

1. Physiotherapy including postural drainage (see Chapter 43)
2. Antibiotics – benzyl pencillin 2–4 mega units intravenously q.d.s. (with or without metronidazole) is the drug of choice in primary lung abscess. Other appropriate antibiotics are required for abscess due to tuberculosis, *klebsiella* or *pseudomonas*. Occasionally the antibiotic can be given through a percutaneous cannula inserted into the abscess. Intravenous antibiotics should be given until the clinical state of the patient has improved (usually about a week). An oral pencillin can then be substituted if benzyl pencillin has been effective, and is usually given empirically for 4–6 weeks. Metronidazole should not be continued for more than 3 weeks because of the risk of toxicity

3. Treat any proximal bronchial obstruction e.g. radiotherapy to a proximal bronchial carcinoma
4. Surgical excision is required only:
   a. if the abscess is beyond an operable proximal bronchial carcinoma, or
   b. to remove an underlying cause such as a bronchogenic cyst or sequestrated segment.

If the patient fails to improve, suspect:

1. Incorrect microbiological diagnosis. The abscess could be due to a specific bacterial infection such as *staphylococcus*, *pseudomonas* or tuberculosis, or to a fungal infection
2. That physiotherapy and postural drainage have been insufficient or incorrectly performed
3. That a proximal stenosis has been overlooked
4. That the 'abscess' could really be a cavitating tumour
5. That the patient has developed an empyema or bronchopleural fistula
6. That the patient has developed infective endocarditis or a cerebral abscess

20. LUNG PROBLEMS IN PATIENTS WITH IMPAIRED RESPIRATORY DEFENCES

The problem

A patient with impaired respiratory defences who develops respiratory symptoms with or without an abnormal chest X-ray.

Types of impairment of respiratory defences

Although this chapter deals mainly with respiratory problems associated with defects of immunity, it is important to remember that factors other than immunity may impair respiratory defences (Table 20.1).

Table 20.1 Types of impairment of respiratory defences

Defects of immunity

        Primary — rare in adults

        Secondary —in some patients with leukaemia, lymphoma, widespread malignancy, immunosuppressive therapy, corticosteroid therapy, irradiation, 'AIDS'.

        (The defect may be of humoral or cellular immunity or in circulatory white cells or in any combination of these)

Underlying lung disease e.g. Chronic bronchitis
                     Bronchiectasis
                     Cystic fibrosis
                     'Immotile cilia'

Metabolic disorders e.g. Severe diabetes
                     Renal failure
                     Hepatic failure

Mechanical e.g. Inability to cough
             Tracheostomy

AN APPROACH TO DIAGNOSIS

Both non-infective and infective conditions must be considered.

Non infective conditions

Although these patients are susceptible to infections with common or uncommon organisms they also develop non-infective conditions related or unrelated to their underlying disease.

— *Pulmonary infarction.* Sick and immobile patients are particularly at risk. Three types of infarcts occur: non-infected emboli from peripheral venous sites, septic emboli (from infected peripheral veins or arterio-venous shunts) or thrombosis due to direct invasion of intrapulmonary vessels by fungus infection

— *Pulmonary oedema* may be due to any of the usual causes or may result from over- enthusiastic or inappropriate intravenous therapy

— *'Shock lung'* may follow a period of hypotension or septicaemia and produces increasing breathlessness with bilateral but perhaps asymmetrical pulmonary shadowing

— *Pulmonary haemorrhage* may complicate thrombocytopenia or anticoagulant therapy or may be a feature of the underlying disease (e.g. Wegener's granuloma or Goodpasture's syndrome). Localised or widespread areas of consolidation which resolve more quickly than would be expected in infection will raise suspicion of pulmonary haemorrhage. Haemoptysis does not necessarily occur

— *Drug reactions.* Diffuse shadowing may result from cytotoxic drugs and diffuse or patchy shadowing with or without blood eosinophilia from many other drugs (see Chapter 35)

— *Extension of the primary disease.* Lymphoma or leukaemia may involve the lung producing a variety of radiological appearances. Lung metastases from solid tumours are usually easily recognisable but lobar or segmental opacities may result from endobronchial metastases or from compression of a bronchus by malignant lymph nodes

— *Irradiation effects.* X-ray shadowing in a recently irradiated area of lung will arouse suspicion.

Infections

— Bacterial. Usual respiratory pathogens. Do not forget that patients with impaired respiratory defences are no less likely than others to develop the 'usual' respiratory infections such as pneumococcal pneumonia, pneumonia complicating chronic bronchitis or influenza, or tuberculosis.

'Opportunist' bacterial infections with organisms which are of low pathogenicity or rarely cause infection in healthy subjects. Particularly important are the Gram-negative bacteria

— Fungi or yeasts. *'Pathogenic'* such as actinomycosis, nocardia, cryptococcus – which are pathogenic to subjects with normal defences. *'Opportunist'* such as candida, aspergillus.

mucormycosis – which are rarely pathogenic in subjects with normal defences
— *Viruses*. Cytomegalovirus (CMV), or Herpes virus infection are the most common
— *Protozoa* especially *Pneumocystis carini* and *Toxoplasma gondii*.

A PRACTICAL APPROACH TO MANAGEMENT

1. **Consider possible non-infective explanations** for symptoms and X-ray changes
2. **If infection seems likely:**
   a. Consider 'usual' infections unrelated to the defect of host defence (influenza, acute bronchitis, pneumococcal pneumonia, etc)
   b. Try to predict the most likely type of opportunist infection from:
      (i) *The clinical state of the patient:*
         — Acute onset with fever in a patient who is 'toxic' suggests bacterial infection.
         — A less acute onset and slow progression suggests fungal infection.
         — The patient who is relatively well but with pulmonary shadowing may have tuberculosis.
         — Breathlessness and a tendency to cough on deep inspiration suggests pneumocystis
      (ii) *The underlying disease.*
         — Acute leukaemia – bacterial infection most common.
         — Lymphoma – fungal infections and tuberculosis are common but bacterial infection occurs if there is neutropenia as a result of therapy.
         — Organ transplantation may be followed by any type of infection. Fungal and bacterial infections are particularly likely after treatment of episodes of rejection with high doses of steroids. Recent advances in immunosuppression therapy with less need for high doses of steroids have reduced the incidence of infective complications
         — Acquired immune deficiency syndrome ('AIDS') is commonly complicated by pneumocystis pneumonia.
      (iii) *The X-ray appearance:*
         — Lobar or segmental consolidation suggests bacterial infection or legionella
         — Single or multiple nodules with or without cavitation suggest fungal or staphylococcal infection

— Consolidation with cavitation suggests fungus infection, staphylococcal, pseudomonas or proteus pneumonia or tuberculosis
— Diffuse bilateral ill-defined shadowing suggests pneumocystis infection, a drug reaction or pulmonary haemorrhage
— Miliary shadowing or upper zone shadowing, especially if also pulmonary or hilar calcification, suggests tuberculosis
— Widespread nodular shadowing suggests cytomegalovirus pneumonia.

(iv) *The peripheral blood count.* Neutropenia predisposes particularly to bacterial or aspergillus infection.
Note: Remember that severely compromised patients may be simultaneously or sequentially infected with several different organisms

3. **Initial laboratory investigations.** Send sputum to the laboratory with specific request that it be stained for tubercle bacilli and examined for fungi as well as bacteria. Collect blood for culture and for serological studies.

The results of sputum examination may be misleading as bacteria, yeasts and fungi may reach sputum from the upper respiratory tract. The repeated presence of aspergillus in the sputum suggests, but does not prove, pulmonary infection. Observation of probable tubercle bacilli is, however, a sufficient basis for starting treatment

4. **Initial decision on management.** A decision must now be made whether to start treatment for the most likely treatable infection or to delay treatment while investigating further. The decision will depend upon the condition of the patient, the rate of the progression of illness and the likelihood of a correct guess at the infecting organism or organisms. We believe that the temptation to treat with antibacterial drugs at this stage should usually be resisted and that every attempt should be made to identify the infecting organism. The results of treating patients with opportunist infection with a 'broad spectrum' of antibacterial agents (often also with high dose cotrimoxazole to 'cover' pneumocystis) are disappointing with the possible exception of severe infection in patients with acute leukaemia

5. **Further attempts to identify infecting agent.** These involve examining bronchial secretions or lung tissue (see footnote):

FOOTNOTE
Meticulous precautions are necessary to protect the operator and other staff if the patient has known or suspected 'AIDS'. Seek expert advice before attempting investigation of such patients.

a. *Transtracheal aspiration* (see Chapter 13) enables bronchial secretions to be collected uncontaminated from the upper respiratory tract

b. *Bronchoscopy*. The fibreoptic bronchoscope allows collection of bronchial secretions either directly or with catheters or brushes passed through the bronchoscope, but the tip of the bronchoscope and the specimens collected are unavoidably contaminated with upper respiratory tract organisms during passage through the nose and pharynx. Specially designed brushes avoid upper respiratory contamination of specimens obtained from the peripheral bronchial tree. Saline can be instilled through the bronchoscope and sucked back. Such 'washings' can be examined for bacteria, fungi, tubercle bacilli or pneumocystis or for macrophages containing haemosiderin from patients with pulmonary haemorrhage.

c. *Biopsy of the lung*. Lung biopsy may be necessary to reach a diagnosis. The available methods are described in Chapter 11. In general transbronchial biopsy is preferred for diffuse shadowing or lobar consolidation and percutaneous biopsy for localised opacities. Biopsy material should be sent for microbiological as well as histological or cytological examination. It is essential that the histologist, cytologist and microbiologist who will receive specimens are aware in advance of the clinical problem and of the diagnostic possibilities so that special stains, examinations or culture methods can be used if needed.

Transbronchial biopsy through the fibreoptic bronchoscope can be accompanied by aspiration of secretions, bronchial washing or bronchial brushing. Possible upper respiratory contamination of specimens does not cause problems in diagnosis of tuberculosis, cytomegalovirus or pneumocystis infection and transbronchial biopsy gives a good yield in these conditions. Biopsies may reveal involvement of the lungs by lymphoma, leukaemia or other malignancies or changes which support drug induced lung damage.

Percutaneous biopsy techniques may be preferable if fungal or bacterial infection is suspected and upper respiratory contamination of specimens must be avoided. The risk of pneumothorax must, however, be taken into account.

Open surgical biopsy may be necessary if other methods have failed to establish a diagnosis and may be the least hazardous method in the presence of a severe bleeding tendency.

Before lung biopsy by any method:
— Measure platelet numbers – if below 50 000 fresh
platelet transfusion may be necessary
— Measure prothrombin time – if prolonged attempt
correction with vitamin K
— Obtain cross-matched blood if haemorrhage is
considered likely
or treat if pulmonary haemorrhage or haemothorax
occurs.

FAILURE TO RESPOND TO TREATMENT

If apparently appropriate chemotherapy for an infection fails to bring
about the hoped-for clinical and radiological improvement the following
possibilities should be considered:
— The organism previously identified may not have been the
cause of respiratory illness (e.g. bacteria or candida isolated
from sputum may have originated from the pharynx and be
unrelated to the lung lesion)
— Two or more different agents may be involved. Bacteria,
fungi and viruses may coexist in the lung lesions of severely
immune deficient patients and treatment of all responsible
agents may be necessary to bring about improvement
— One or more additional factors may be important (e.g. an
obstructed bronchus, repeated pulmonary emboli, a
developing empyema).
The original investigations may have to be repeated or additional tests
carried out. Increasingly frenzied addition of further anti-microbial drugs
without a microbiological diagnosis is rarely successful and exposes the
patient to the hazards of drug toxicity.

21. TUBERCULOSIS

The prevalence of tuberculosis in the Western world has been falling for many years (in the UK the number of newly recognised cases halves every 5 years). Because of its supposed 'disappearance' failure to consider a diagnosis of tuberculosis is all too often the cause of delays in treatment, or even the death of the patient. Physicians should be aware of the local epidemiology of tuberculosis in the region in which they work. For example throughout the UK most new cases are elderly British-born men, but in areas with large numbers of Asian immigrants the disease, often in an unusual form, occurs predominantly in the immigrant population.

Consider tuberculosis in an adult with:
— Persisting cough of recent onset, or worsening of a chronic cough
— haemoptysis
— weight loss
— pleural effusion

With the exception of patients with pleural effusion there may be no abnormality detectable on clinical examination of the chest even in the presence of quite extensive tuberculosis.

All such patients should have a chest X-ray. A normal chest X-ray virtually excludes the diagnosis of pulmonary tuberculosis. Abnormalities which should alert one to the possibility of tuberculosis are:
— patchy shadowing in the upper lobes
— cavitation in the apical segments of upper or lower lobes
— shrinkage of one or both upper lobes
— calcified opacities in the lung or in mediastinal lymph nodes
— enlarged intrathoracic lymph nodes in a child or someone of Asian stock
— pleural effusion
— widespread miliary shadowing

INVESTIGATIONS TO CONFIRM OR EXCLUDE TUBERCULOSIS

ESR

This time-honoured test is of no practical value in diagnosis of tuberculosis. A raised ESR may have innumerable other causes and a low value does not exclude active tuberculosis.

Examination of sputum

Several specimens of sputum (not saliva!) should be sent to the laboratory with a specific request that they be examined for *M. tuberculosis*. Many microbiology laboratories no longer routinely examine all specimens for tubercle bacilli unless specifically asked to do so. At least three specimens should be examined because the number of organisms may vary from time to time, individual cultures may become contaminated in the laboratory, and recognition of acid-alcohol fast bacilli in several specimens provides more convincing evidence of tuberculosis than occasional organisms in just one specimen.

Stained smears of sputum

A report of 'No organism seen' may indicate that:
1. and unsatisfactory specimen was sent
2. insufficient numbers of tubercle bacilli were present in that specimen to be seen on microscopy although the patient does have tuberculosis
3. the patient does not have active pulmonary tuberculosis.

Cultures

Cultures may be available between 3 and 8 weeks. Positive cultures nearly always indicate tuberculosis but the possibility of infection with other mycobacteria must be borne in mind. The microbiologist can at this stage do no more than report the presence or absence of organisms 'having the cultural characteristics of *M. tuberculosis*'. Identification of the type of mycobacterium must await further laboratory study. Negative cultures after 8 weeks from a patient who is not receiving antituberculous therapy means either that unsatisfactory samples have been examined or that no viable tubercle bacilli were present at the time of sputum collection.

The likelihood that a patient with pulmonary tuberculosis will excrete bacilli in the sputum varies with the type and stage of disease. In the presence of pneumonic shadowing, cavitation or severe symptoms large numbers of bacilli in the sputum would be anticipated and if none are found an alternative diagnosis should be sought. On the other hand, patients with lobar shrinkage, calcified opacities or single opacities are much less likely to shed tubercle bacilli in sputum even if their disease is tuberculous and negative cultures do not necessarily cast doubt on the tuberculous origin of the abnormality (but do suggest that they are unlikely to infect others).

Interpretation of the chest X-ray

The activity and infectivity of tuberculosis cannot be reliably judged from X-ray appearances. Thus a patient who is known to have had long-standing fibrosis of an upper lobe which has not changed radiographically for some years may nevertheless be shedding tubercle bacilli and may infect others. Cavitation or increasing lung shadowing suggest active disease. Reduced volume of a lobe or lobes usually represents fibrosis (i.e. long-standing disease) or less often tuberculous bronchostenosis. Calcification likewise indicates long-standing disease but evidence of 'old' tuberculous infection does not exclude currently active and infective disease.

Enlargement of intrathoracic lymph nodes is uncommon in white adults with tuberculosis (but does occur in children) but is common amongst Asians in whom it may or may not be associated with pulmonary shadows. If enlarged intrathoracic lymph nodes are due to tuberculosis the disease must be assumed to be active and to require treatment.

The tuberculin skin test

This test, though it may provide additional evidence, cannot in itself be used to confirm or exclude a diagnosis of tuberculosis. Interpretation of these tests is discussed in Chapter 15.

Other methods of investigation

Other methods of obtaining diagnostic material are available if no sputum can be obtained

— Bronchoscopy (usually with the fibreoptic instrument) has superseded the previous techniques of laryngeal swabs or gastric aspirate. In patients in whom pulmonary tuberculosis is suspected but from whose sputum no tubercle bacilli can be obtained, bronchoscopy allows aspiration of secretions from the abnormal portion of lung and biopsy of bronchial mucosa or of lung. The specimens are stained and cultured for mycobacteria, and histological examination of biopsy tissue may confirm the diagnosis or reveal an alternative cause of the pulmonary shadowing. Bronchoscopy should not be undertaken without careful thought in such patients because of the small, but real, risk of exposing those carrying out the procedure to infection

— Enlarged mediastinal lymph nodes may be accessible to biopsy at mediastinoscopy but biopsy may require anterior mediastinotomy or thoracotomy

— Pleural biopsy and examination of pleural fluid in tuberculous pleural effusion are discussed in Chapter 27.

MANAGEMENT OF TUBERCULOSIS

The success of treatment depends upon regular administration of effective combinations of anti-tuberculous drugs. Different regimens of chemotherapy have been extensively studied and it is irresponsible and unnecessary to prescribe unconventional drug combinations or dosages without good reason. Although modern drug regimens may appear simple to prescribe, failure of treatment is still most often the result of incorrect prescribing or lack of awareness of the best methods of assessing response and ensuring patient co-operation. The chemotherapy of tuberculosis should follow the same principles and regimens for all sites of disease (with the exception of meningitis). Traditional forms of treatment such as bed rest or special diets do not improve the response to antituberculous drugs.

Anti-tuberculous drugs

Several effective combinations of anti-tuberculous drugs for treatment of newly diagnosed tuberculosis are in use. They have in common an initial phase of 2 months of treatment with 3 or 4 drugs to rapidly reduce the bacterial population and to avoid failure of treatment should the organisms be resistant to one of the drugs.

A highly effective regimen comprises 9 months of therapy as follows: 2 months of rifampicin, isoniazid and ethambutol followed by 7 months of isoniazid and rifampicin. Pyrazinamide is a satisfactory alternative to ethambutol in this regimen.

Recent evidence indicates that a 6 month course of treatment starting with 4 drugs is effective as follows: 2 months rifampicin, isoniazid, ethambutol and pyrazinamide followed by 4 months of rifampicin and isoniazid.

In order to prevent the uncommon but important side effect of peripheral neuropathy due to isoniazid, pyridoxine 10 mg daily may be prescribed throughout therapy to those at particular risk (elderly, malnourished, pregnant, chronic liver disease).

Dosages

Rifampacin – 600 mg daily for a subject over 50 kg bodyweight, 450 mg daily under this weight.

Isoniazid – 300 mg daily.

Ethambutol – 15 mg per kg body weight (most of the published trials used 25 mg per kg bodyweight for the first 2 months of therapy but this carries a higher risk of ocular toxicity and has not been shown to be superior to 15 mg/kg).

Pyrazinamide – 1.5 g daily if under 50 kg, 2 g daily if 50 to 60 kg, 2.5 g daily if over 70 kg.

Anti-tuberculous drugs are most effective if administered as a single daily dose which is easier for the patient to remember. Dosages may need to be reduced in patients with renal failure or severe liver disease.

Several of these drugs are available in combination tablets which are preferred, not only to minimise the number of tablets prescribed, but also to reduce the likelihood of the patient erroneously taking a single drug. Combinations of rifampicin with isoniazid and of ethambutol with isoniazid are available at different doses and enable the correct daily dosage to be given.

Adverse effects from anti-tuberculous drugs

Most patients suffer no serious or troublesome adverse effects from modern anti-tuberculous drugs but some side effects may be serious, disabling or even fatal. The commonest side effects are listed below.

Rifampicin

Nausea with abdominal pain or anorexia may occur but are uncommon. Although rises of serum transaminase levels are common during the early weeks of treatment clinically important hepatitis is rare. It is not helpful to perform regular liver function tests unless there is pre-existing liver disease but treatment must be stopped immediately if jaundice or other symptoms of liver dysfunction such as nausea or severe anorexia occur. Less common side effects include febrile flu-like reactions (more common if the drug is taken intermittently), thrombocytopenia or abdominal pain. Rifampicin induces liver enzymes and doses of corticosteroids, anticoagulants, oral hypoglycaemic agents and digitalis may need to be increased at the onset of treatment and, very important, decreased again when rifampicin therapy stops. Oral contraceptive drugs become less effective during rifampicin therapy and alternative methods of contraception should be advised.

Isoniazid

Peripheral neuropathy is uncommon at the dosage recommended but can be prevented by a small regular dose of pyridoxine. Hepatitis is uncommon but may be serious. Hypersensitivity reaction with rash and fever are uncommon.

Ethambutol

The most serious side effect is optic neuritis. This occurs only with doses higher than 15 mg per kg or in the presence of impaired renal function. With doses of 15 mg per kg we do not believe it necessary to test visual acuity during therapy but patients should be warned of the small risk of visual symptoms and questioned about possible visual side effects during therapy. If patients develop any visual symptoms ethambutol must be stopped until an expert ophthalmic opinion has been obtained.

Pyrazinamide

When previously used in high dosage in combination with other toxic drugs acquired a reputation for toxicity. More recent studies show infrequent side effects, mainly fever and arthralgia. Although pyrazinamide may be hepatotoxic at high dose this is uncommon at the doses now used. Serum uric acid consistently rises early in treatment but gout is uncommon.

PRACTICAL ASPECTS OF TREATING TUBERCULOSIS

Infectiousness

A patient with pulmonary tuberculosis can infect others only by disseminating infected droplets whilst coughing. Infection is not spread by talking or just by personal contact. The patient who does not cough is unlikely to infect others. A patient whose sputum contains too few organisms to be seen on microscopy is of very low infectivity and represents a negligible hazard to the community. Within 2–3 weeks of starting modern anti-tuberculous therapy patients are probably no longer infectious even though organisms (which are probably dead) may still be seen in stained specimens of the sputum. *Barrier nursing and the wearing of masks and gowns by medical or nursing staff does not protect against infection and is not necessary.* Patients must be encouraged to cough into sputum cartons and if the cough is uncontrolled the patient should wear a mask. The domestic dishwasher will kill any mycobacteria present on eating utensils and special cutlery and utensils are not necessary. Urine and faeces are not infectious. Infection is not transmitted by organisms on personal belongings, books or other articles. Bedding can be washed or laundered in the usual way.

Place of treatment

Most patients can be treated at home unless they are ill enough to require nursing care or cannot be relied upon to take chemotherapy regularly or are unavoidably exposed to young children at home. It is no longer justifiable to confine all patients to hospital solely to protect the community. Even highly infectious patients may be treated at home if they avoid contact with young children and with people outside their immediate family. Members of the family (with the exception of infants and young children) are unlikely to become infected after the diagnosis of tuberculosis has been made if they have escaped infection previously. If hospital treatment is required a single room in a general hospital is suitable and the patient should wear a mask when leaving the room during the first 2 weeks of therapy. After use the room should be vacated and aired for 24 hours and, after conventional cleaning, is then safe for other patients.

Non-compliant patients

Several regimes of fully supervised therapy have been shown to be effective and are recommended for patients who are unlikely to conform to regular self treatment. After an initial *fully supervised* 2 month course of daily combined oral treatment, possibly in hospital (see above), therapy may be continued with twice weekly supervised drug administration. Each dose may comprise either isoniazid orally at the high dose of 14 mg/kg (900 mg for an average adult), with streptomycin 1 g intramuscularly, or isoniazid at this high dose with rifampicin 600 mg orally. It is wise to continue such intermittent regimens for 1 year. Careful supervision of every dose is essential and it is not sufficient merely to give unreliable patients their tablets on the assumption, or with the assurance, that they will be swallowed. Intermittent rifampicin therapy carries a higher risk of toxicity than daily treatment including a flu-like syndrome, haemolysis or thrombocytopenia.

Supervision of chemotherapy

Anti-tuberculous drugs are effective only if taken regularly and in correct dosage. Many patients are tempted to reduce the frequency or dosage of their drugs as they begin to feel better and all should be warned of the hazards of doing so. Many methods of testing compliance have been studied but, rightly or wrongly, few chest physicians apply these as a routine. Regular supervision by a physician who is aware of this problem and in whom the patient has trust is probably as satisfactory a way of ensuring regular treatment as any. The elderly and ill may be forgetful and drug therapy should therefore be simplified as much as possible, bottles clearly labelled, and relatives or friends enrolled to remind the patient of the need for regular treatment.

Observations during therapy

Regular supervision is required to monitor progress of the disease, ensure that therapy is being taken and to detect adverse effects. Progress of the disease is best assessed by serial examination of sputum for tubercle bacilli. In the early weeks of therapy organisms may still be seen on stained smears but the numbers of organisms should be falling and cultures should become negative well before 3 months. It is essential that sputum, if available, is cultured regularly during chemotherapy and at the end of treatment. Changes in the chest X-ray are of less importance than examination of sputum. It is expected that recent shadows will resolve, often without residual fibrosis, but there will be no change in already fibrotic or calcified lesions. Cavities usually close but failure to do so is not a cause of anxiety if sputum no longer contains organisms. Persisting cavities may, however, become colonised with aspergillus with the development of a mycetoma.

Failure to respond to treatment

If large numbers of organisms persist on stained smears or if cultures remain positive it is likely that the patient has not been taking the drugs as recommended. Primary drug resistance of *M. tuberculosis* in patients who have not received previous treatment is very uncommon in developed countries and even if present should not result in failure of therapy if combined drugs have been given. In practice clinical, bacteriological and radiographic improvement has usually occurred by the time the results of antibiotic sensitivity are available from sputa collected at the onset, and it is usually unnecessary to change chemotherapy even if drug resistance is reported.

Follow-up after completion of chemotherapy

The great majority of patients who complete a full course of anti-tuberculous therapy with bacteriological and radiographic improvement have been cured of their disease. Relapse when it occurs is usually apparent within 1 year of the end of treatment. It is therefore our policy to discharge otherwise fit patients from follow-up at this time if we belive that they are likely to have taken chemotherapy as recommended. Relapse whether it occurs after an inadequate duration of chemotherapy or after a full course is usually due to organisms which are still sensitive to the standard drugs.

Examination of contacts

This has two purposes, namely to identify the source of infection and to identify those who might have acquired infection from the patient. In the UK responsibility for examination of contacts rests with Community Physicians in collaboration with chest physicians and only broad principles will be discussed here. It must be remembered that Community Physicians can be aware of cases of tuberculosis and the need for surveillance of contacts only if index cases are notified to them.

In an attempt to find the source of infection all adult members of the family of a child or young person with tuberculosis of any type should have a chest X-ray as should school teachers and others in regular contact if no family source can be found. It is rarely possible to find the source from which an adult has been infected, but domestic contacts should anyhow be checked.

Domestic contacts of those with infectious tuberculosis should have a chest X-ray if adult, or tuberculin test if children. Chest X-rays, if normal, should be repeated in 6 months and 1 year, and in the case of Asians in 2 years. Children who show a negative tuberculin test soon after tuberculosis has been diagnosed in a contact, should have the test repeated 2 months after the last exposure. The risk of transmission of infection to contacts other than family, household members or close friends is small and it is not usually recommended that workmates and casual contacts are investigated. Patients with repeatedly negative sputum cultures or with non-pulmonary tuberculosis are of very low infectivity.

Mycobacteria other than M. tuberculosis

Infection with these so called 'atypical', 'anomymous' or saprophytic mycobacteria are uncommon in the UK. The diagnosis rests on identification of organisms isolated from sputum or other materials. Investigation and management is usually the province of the specialised Chest Physician and will not be considered here.

Chemoprophylaxis

Almost the only situation in which 'primary chemoprophylaxis' is now used (the administration of anti-tuberculous drugs to an individual who has not previously been infected), is to protect a newborn baby who is breast-fed by an infectious tuberculous mother.

'Secondary prophylaxis' consists of giving anti-tuberculous drugs to an individual whose only evidence of infection is a positive tuberculin skin test. This is justified in infants and in children under 5 because of the knowledge that infection has been recent and because of the known significant risk of development of tuberculous disease. We do not believe that chemoprophylaxis is justified in school children found to be tuberculin positive at routine testing at the age of 12. Children, and indeed adolescents, from the Indian subcontinent have a much greater risk of developing active disease and should be offered chemoprophylaxis if they are tuberculin positive. Children who have been recent contacts of a case of pulmonary tuberculosis and who are tuberculin positive should be offered chemoprophylaxis.

This is the only situation in which one drug is sufficient and isoniazid in an adult dosage of 300 mg daily for 12 months is effective. The risks of poor compliance in this situation are self-evident.

Prevention of reactivation of previous tuberculosis

Patients with previous pulmonary or extrathoracic tuberculosis who have never received anti-tuberculous drugs are at risk of reactivation of disease. A course of anti-tuberculous therapy with modern drugs to eradicate residual bacteria and remove, or very greatly reduce, the risk of reactivation in future years is often recommended. On public health grounds alone the benefits of treating such patients are self-evident for this group is responsible for much of the spread of tuberculous infection in the community. For the individual, however, the decision is more difficult and the risks of adverse effects from chemotherapy and of poor compliance must be weighed carefully against the risks of reactivation of disease which, unfortunately, cannot be quantified. In this situation we recommend at least two anti-tuberculous drugs for at least 9 months.

Extrathoracic tuberculosis

Tuberculosis of lymph nodes

The commonest site of extrathoracic lymph node tuberculosis is the cervical chain. Nearly all such infections are now caused by *M. tuberculosis* of human strain but a few are due to atypical mycobacteria or rarely bovine mycobacterium. Tuberculosis of lymph nodes is more common amongst those from the Indian subcontinent where it may be suspected from the association of enlarged, possibly fluctuant, lymph nodes in a patient who is otherwise not apparently ill and who has a strongly positive tuberculin skin test. Under these circumstances confirmation of the diagnosis by removal of nodes or aspiration may be considered unnecessary. The diagnosis is likely if calcification is seen in lymph nodes on X-ray indicating previous tuberculosis but biopsy or excision of nodes may be necessary to confirm the diagnosis.

Treatment follows the scheme and dosage for pulmonary tuberculosis and the response to modern treatment is excellent although episodes of enlargement or fluctuation of nodes may develop during the course of therapy. Unless symptoms are severe surgical drainage or excision is rarely required and most such patients will eventually be cured by continued chemotherapy. In the absence of clinical trials on shorter courses of treatment eighteen months of drugs is advised.

Renal tuberculosis

The diagnosis is suspected in patients with sterile pyuria or with haematuria or persisting dysuria and is confirmed by culture of *M. tuberculosis* from urine. The response to the scheme of anti-tuberculous therapy used for pulmonary tuberculosis is usually excellent and nephrectomy or surgical intervention is required only if the kidney has been severely damaged or if a large abscess is present. If ureteric obstruction is present or develops during treatment prednisolone 20 mg daily is added to the anti-tuberculous regimen.

Tuberculous meningitis

Tuberculous meningitis, though now uncommon in developed countries, still carries a very high mortality in part due to delayed diagnosis. It may occur as an apparently isolated event or in association with miliary tuberculosis. Even with modern anti-tuberculous chemotherapy the mortality and residual morbidity remains high. No adequately controlled studies of chemotherapy are available but it is probably wise to start treatment with intramuscular streptomycin, and oral rifampicin, isoniazid, ethambutol and pyrazinamide. Additional intrathecal streptomycin increases the risk of eighth nerve toxicity and there is no evidence that it improves the response to modern therapy. The role of corticosteroids remains controversial. Intramuscular streptomycin is given in the dose of 1 g daily if renal function is normal (0.75 g daily in a patient who is over 40). Isoniazid is given in the high dose of 15 mg/kg bodyweight. Ethambutol is used at a dose of 25 mg/kg but is best avoided if the patient is too young or too ill to report visual loss.

BCG immunisation

BCG immunisation is still widely used in the UK and in Europe but less so in the USA. As the prevalence of tuberculosis falls the place of BCG immunisation is constantly under review. Freeze-dried vaccine is stable when stored at the correct temperature. 0.1 ml of vaccine is administered by intradermal injection over the insertion of the deltoid to raise a weal (injection too near the tip of the shoulder may result in ulceration and scarring). When large numbers are to be immunised multiple puncture instruments are used for convenience. It is not easy to correctly administer an intradermal injection by needle and syringe particularly to a frightened child. Such injections should be given by those who are experienced and have been trained, as subdermal administration of BCG may cause an abscess to form. 3–4 weeks after innoculation a papule appears which may persist for several weeks and may occasionally ulcerate and discharge. The axillary lymph nodes may become slightly tender and enlarged. Complications are uncommon. A local abscess or pain and swelling of axillary nodes usually represents low grade secondary bacterial infection and responds to an antibiotic such as erythromycin. A persisting cold abscess or ulcer may develop at the site of injection. This usually subsides without treatment but may very occasionally require a short course of isoniazid by mouth if there is no response to 2 weeks of treatment with erythromycin. The only contraindications to BCG immunisation are severe immune deficiency, local sepsis or eczema, a known positive tuberculin skin test, and innoculation with another live vaccine (except oral poliomyelitis vaccine) within 3 weeks.

Policies for BCG immunisation vary widely from country to country. In the UK children receive a tuberculin test at the age of about 12 and BCG is administered to those with negative or grade 1 Heaf reactions. BCG is administered at birth or in infancy to those at special risk of acquiring infection from their environment, including all newborn babies of immigrants from India and Pakistan. It is also given to those at risk of exposure to tuberculosis such as nurses, doctors, medical laboratory technicians, others who work closely with patients in hospitals and children who are travelling to countries in which tuberculosis is common.

22. BRONCHIECTASIS

Bronchiectasis is the persistent dilatation of bronchi. The various descriptive terms such as cylindrical, fusiform and saccular bronchiectasis are of little clinical importance.

Effect of bronchiectasis

The effect of broncheictasis depends on several factors.

Site
Bronchial secretions are poorly cleared from dilated bronchi in dependent parts of the lung but do not accumulate in upper parts of the lung from which they drain spontaneously by gravity. Hence sputum is common with lower lobe but uncommon with upper lobe bronchiectasis.

Extent
Bronchiectasis of one or two lobes may cause no breathlessness if the remaining lung is normal. Airflow obstruction is common in patients with widespread bronchiectasis, often with hypoxaemia which can in turn lead to pulmonary hypertension and right heart failure.

Infection
Infection, usually occurring with upper respiratory organisms, is a sequel to stasis of secretions.

Bleeding
This may be slight from inflamed bronchial mucosa or heavy from dilated bronchial arteries (which contain blood at systemic pressure).

Diagnosis

Consider bronchiectasis in a patient with:
- Persistent cough with purulent sputum which is often worse on change of posture
- Episodic cough with purulent sputum which often occurs after upper respiratory infection
- Haemoptysis, especially in patients with symptoms of 1 or 2 above
- Recurrent pneumonia involving the same part of the lung
- Recurrent pleuritic pain in the same site.

Examination

On examination there may be:
- *No detectable abnormality*, if bronchiectasis is localised, especially if there is little accumulation of secretions
- *Inspiratory crackles*; early and mid-inspiratory crackles are heard over the affected part of the lung, often with additional coarser sounds of secretions in the larger airways. These latter sounds may change or clear after coughing and may be heard also during expiration
- *Clubbing of fingers*, if bronchiectasis is widespread and chronically infected
- *Central cyanosis*, if bronchiectasis is widespread
- *Right heart failure* which may develop if bronchiectasis is widespread.

Causes to consider

- Previous pneumonia or bronchiolitis in childhood – often complicating whooping cough or measles (causing localised or widespread bronchiectasis)
- Previous pneumonia in adult life especially if slow to resolve or if complicated by lung abscess or empyema (usually causes localised bronchiectasis)
- Tuberculosis with residual fibrosis of affected lung (usually upper lobes) or with residual collapse and bronchiectasis of middle lobe as a sequeal to lymph node compression of this bronchus
- Bronchial obstruction or narrowing which may result from inhaled foreign body (often right lower lobe); bronchial tumour or stricture
- Aspiration – repeated inhalation of gastro-oesophageal contents or of food (usually lower lobes or dependent parts of lung)
- Congenital disorders – cystic fibrosis (see Chapter 23); immotile cilia (with or without situs inversus, and other features of Kartagener's syndrome); developmental abnormalities such as bronchial atresia or pulmonary sequestration
- Allergic bronchopulmonary aspergillosis – usually in patients with asthma (often causes bronchiectasis in upper lobes)
- With systemic diseases:
  a. Generalised immune deficiency especially congenital or acquired gamma globulin deficiency
  b. Rheumatoid disease
  c. Inflammatory bowel disease, (ulcerative colitis or Crohn's disease)
  d. Syndrome of yellow nails and lymphoedema.

Investigations

Chest X-ray
This may show:
- No abnormality in patients with small areas of bronchiectasis, especially if there is little retention of secretions
- Loss of volume of one or more lobes or segments with or without shadowing due to fibrosis or associated pneumonia, or calcification suggestive of previous tuberculosis
- Dilated bronchi – seen end-on as small ring shadows and side-on as parallel lines ('tram-lines'), or, if filled with secretions, as tubular shadows
- Dextrocardia of Kartagener's syndrome
- Secondary cardiovascular effects of pulmonary hypertension (dilated proximal pulmonary arteries, cardiac enlargement).

Bronchogram
A bronchogram is usually not required for diagnosis if there is a characteristic history and if the plain chest X-ray shows changes consistent with bronchiectasis.

A bronchogram is required only if:
- there is doubt about the diagnosis
- surgical resection is being considered
- knowledge of exact site of bronchiectasis will improve efficiency of postural drainage.

It is unwise to perform bronchography if a patient:
- is breathless, cyanosed or has heart failure because the procedure then carries a risk
- has recently had an increase in sputum, because retained secretions may impair filling of bronchi with contrast medium
- has recently had pneumonia, because dilatation of bronchi may occur for weeks or months after pneumonia, only to revert to normal later ('reversible bronchiectasis').

Other possible investigations
To investigate the cause of bronchiectasis the following may be helpful (if other features suggest these possibilities):
- Sweat test – for cystic fibrosis in younger patients with bilateral disease
- Serum immunoglobulins – for immune deficiency
- Skin test and tests for precipitins – for allergic bronchopulmonary aspergillosis
- Barium swallow – for swallowing defect or gastro-oesophageal aspiration
- Sputum – for tubercle bacilli
- Biopsy of nasal mucosa – to study motility of cilia or for electron microscopy – for immotile cilia syndrome
- Lymphogram – for yellow nail syndrome and lymphoedema.

To assess the severity of bronchiectasis the following may be helpful
 — Spirometry – to measure loss of ventilatory function (both airflow obstruction and restrictive defect may occur)
 — Arterial blood gases – low Po_2 or raised Pco_2 indicate severe and extensive disease
 — Blood count – polycythaemia may be a response to chronic hypoxaemia. Leucocytosis is uncommon even during episodes of purulent sputum
 — ECG – is abnormal only as a result of pulmonary hypertension.

As a guide to treatment:
 — Sputum examination is often not helpful as a guide to antibiotic therapy and frequently no recognised pathogens are found even from purulent sputum. Examination for tubercle bacilli is essential if the history or X-ray suggest previous tuberculosis.
 — A bronchogram may occasionally be useful in planning postural drainage.

Management

 — *Patients with few or no symptoms* require no treatment
 — *Patients with recurrent cough and sputum*
   a. Physiotherapy (see Chapter 43). Postural drainage and 'huffing' to aid clearance of bronchial secretions should be taught initially by a physiotherapist and can then be carried out by the patient at home (with or without the aid of a member of the family)
   b. Antibiotics in short courses may speed clearing of purulent sputum but sputum often becomes mucoid after postural drainage alone. Choice of antibiotic is as for treatment of purulent exacerbation of chronic bronchitis (see Chapter 29). Continuous antibiotics whether with one or a sequence of drugs do not prevent exacerbations and are not recommended. It is not known whether antibiotic courses taken at the time of upper respiratory infections prevent development of purulent sputum
   c. Annual influenza immunisation is probably advisable.
 — *Patients with persistent cough and sputum*
   a. Postural drainage and 'huffing' as above should be carried out regularly, once or more each day
   b. Continuous antibiotic therapy is rarely of value but short courses may be given when systemic symptoms occur or when sputum volume or purulence increases. If culture of sputum consistently shows unusual organisms such as pseudomonas special antibiotic regimes may be necessary.

Injections of gammaglobulin may help patients with
immunoglobulin deficiency. Annual influenza immunisation
is desirable.

— *Specific symptoms*

  a. Breathlessness due to airflow obstruction can usually be
improved somewhat by removal of sputum with postural
drainage. Bronchodilator therapy may bring about further
improvement (see Chapter 30). Corticosteroids are rarely of
value

  b. Haemoptysis may cease after antibiotics and postural
drainage if associated with purulent sputum, but is much
more difficult to treat if it occurs without sputum.
Occasionally severe haemoptysis requires surgical resection
of the affected lung

  c. Heart failure requires conventional treatment with
diuretics but, as for some patients with severe chronic
bronchitis, long-term domiciliary oxygen therapy may be
considered

  d. Rare complications such as empyema, cerebral abscess or
amyloidosis require appropriate investigation and
treatment.

Surgical resection is rarely necessary but may be considered if
bronchiectasis is confined to one lobe or to adjacent lobes (as shown on
bilateral bronchograms), the rest of the lungs being healthy and

  1. Persistent sputum production or recurrent haemoptysis remain
a problem after prolonged and energetic medical treatment

  2. The underlying cause of the bronchiectasis is no longer
present

23. CYSTIC FIBROSIS IN ADOLESCENTS AND ADULTS

Cystic fibrosis is usually recognised early in childhood but now that 70% of those who have survived infancy live to reach the age of 18, adolescents and adults with cystic fibrosis will increasingly be the responsibility of general and specialised physicians.

Cystic fibrosis is occasionally first recognised in adolescent or adult life, either because long-standing symptoms have been attributed to other conditions such as bronchitis or asthma, or because the symptoms first occurred or were first reported after childhood.

Consider cystic fibrosis when symptoms of bronchiectasis (cough and purulent sputum with or without breathlessness) slowly increase, especially if the disease is bilateral and if either *Staphylococcus pyogenes* or *Pseudomonas aeruginosa* are isolated from sputum. Nasal polyps, weight loss, persisting diarrhoea or bouts of abdominal pain increase the suspicion.

Common symptoms

— Cough with purulent sputum is almost invariable. The sputum may occasionally be streaked with blood.
— Breathlessness is related to the severity of airflow obstruction.

Physical examination

Adolescents and adults with cystic fibrosis are usually of average height but are almost invariably underweight by the time they develop significant symptoms. Clubbing of the fingers and toes is common if there are chest symptoms. Nasal obstruction may be due to polyps. Early inspiratory crackles, with or without an expiratory wheeze, can usually be heard on listening to the chest characteristically in the mid and upper zones.

Confirming the diagnosis

The sweat test

Analysis of sodium concentration of sweat obtained by pilocarpine iontophoresis is the cornerstone of diagnosis in childhood but this test is less reliable in adult life. Sweat sodium concentrations greater than 70 mmol/l are found in about one third of healthy adults and are therefore not diagnosis of cystic fibrosis except in childhood. However a sweat sodium level of less than 50–60 mmol/l eliminates the diagnosis of cystic fibrosis. It has been suggested that the raised sweat sodium concentrations of normal adults may fall after treatment with 9 alpha fluoro hydrocortisone whereas no such reduction occurs in patients with cystic fibrosis, but this is probably not a reliable test.

Misleading results may be obtained unless the sweat test is performed by someone experienced in the technique and a sufficient volume of sweat is analysed by a laboratory where such specimens are regularly handled. An incorrectly performed or analysed test may lead to an eroneous diagnosis of cystic fibrosis with disastrous consequences if this leads to an incorrectly gloomy prognosis. It is unwise to base the diagnosis on a single sweat test and if in any doubt the test should be repeated. It is wise not to make a diagnosis of cystic fibrosis from the sweat test unless sodium concentrations consistently above 90 mmol/l are obtained from more than one sweat sample weighing at least 100 mg (Lower weights may reflect evaporation from the specimen which will raise the concentration of sodium.)

Pancreatic function tests
Faecal fat collection on a normal diet will usually confirm steatorrhoea and duodenal intubation is rarely necessary. Measurement of faecal trypsin is of no value in diagnosis.

Chest X-ray

This may occasionally be normal when the diagnosis is first considered or, in the early stages or mild case, subtle abnormalities such as tubular parallel line shadows may be overlooked. Usually ring shadows representing bronchiectatic airways coexist with patchy shadows mainly in the mid and upper zones. The lungs remain well inflated and, as airflow obstruction increases, over-inflated. The hila may become prominent as pulmonary hypertension develops and the heart may enlarge if cor pulmonale develops.

Other features and complications

Respiratory
— Episodes of increased cough with purulent sputum and worsening breathlessness are common
— Haemoptysis may occur at these times
— Pneumothorax is common and may be difficult to detect in a patient with previously over-inflated lungs and airflow obstruction
— Respiratory failure and congestive heart failure develop late in the course of the disease.

Non-respiratory

— Pancreatic steatorrhea with malabsorption is usually not a
   major problem after childhood
— Cirrhosis with portal hypertension may develop
— 'Meconium ileus equivalent' may cause small bowel
   obstruction or repeated episodes of severe abdominal pain.
   This seems to be due to abnormally solid faeces
— Diabetes mellitus. Reduced glucose tolerance is not
   uncommon but severe diabetes requiring insulin is rare
— Infertility. The genitalia are normal but puberty is delayed.
   Males are almost invariably infertile due to azoospermia and
   this finding supports a diagnosis of cystic fibrosis if this is
   in doubt. Females have reduced fertility but pregnancy may
   occur
— Hypertrophic osteoarthropathy with pain and swelling of
   large joints in association with clubbing.

Assessment

— Sputum is almost invariably purulent. *Staph. pyogenes* may be
   isolated but more commonly in older patients mucoid strains
   of *psuedomonas aeruginosa* are present. *Haemophilus
   influenzae is* less commonly isolated
— Lung function. Airflow obstruction may be measured by
   simple spirometry (remember the potential problem of
   contaminating spirometers with antibiotic-resistant bacteria).
   As the disease progresses arterial blood shows progressive
   hypoxaemia and eventually a rising CO_2 tension
— Liver function tests – serum alkaline phosphatase is
   frequently elevated
— Immunological tests. Approximately half of all patients with
   cystic fibrosis show multiple positive reactions to skin prick
   tests to common allergens. Reactions against *Aspergillus
   fumigatus* are common and precipitins may be found in the
   blood, but clinically recognised episodes of bronchopulmonary
   aspergillosis are uncommon.

MANAGEMENT

In a chronic and invariably fatal condition such as cystic fibrosis,
management must follow a long-term plan and this is best undertaken by
those experienced in treating the disease. Consideration of the effects of the
disease on the emotional, domestic, educational and working life are as
important as other aspects of treatment.

Principles of regular treatment

Respiratory

Removal of secretions
Encouragement to cough (or 'huff') out secretions together with postural drainage are important and should be carried out frequently and regularly.

Antibiotics
Improved survival in cystic fibrosis may, at least in part, be related to better antibiotic therapy in the earlier stages of the disease. Most children receive regular antibiotics but the value of continuous antibiotics in adult life is uncertain.

Bronchodilators
The airflow obstruction in cystic fibrosis may be improved to a varying degree by inhaled bronchodilators. (For principles and details, see Chapter 30). Occasional patients with severe airflow obstruction may benefit from corticosteroids orally or by inhalation and this treatment does not seem to increase the severity or complications of pulmonary infection.

Immunisation
Annual influenza immunisation is a wise precaution.

Exacerbations and complications

Exacerbations of respiratory symptoms

These must be tackled energetically with vigorous physiotherapy to remove secretions. Short courses of oral antibiotics may sometimes produce improvement, the choice depending on the results of sputum culture. Flucloxacillin or erythromycin if *S. pyogenes* is present, amoxicillin for *H. influenzae* or chloramphenicol if several organisms are isolated or if other antibiotics have failed. None of these treatments has much effect on pseudomonas and severe exacerbations require an attempt to tackle this organism. There seems little to choose between various regimes of intravenous therapy with either gentamicin or tobramycin together with carbenicillin. An intravenous 'line' may prevent thrombosis of peripheral veins. Serum levels of gentamicin or tobramycin should be measured to avoid toxicity. Hypokalaemia and sodium overload frequently complicates carbenicillin therapy. Ticaricillin and azlocillin have activity against pseudomonas but seem to offer no great advantage in practice. The 'third generation' cephalosporins are proving valuable. Ceftazidime can be given every 8 hours through an indwelling venous cannula, treatment which can, with the cooperation of parents and family doctor, sometimes be given at home to avoid the need for hospital admission. Ciprofloxacin, an oral antipseudomonas agent, shows promise.

Treatment never eradicates pseudomonas infection but a response can be gauged by reduced purulence of sputum, improvement in general well-being and appetite and a small but useful improvement of FEV_1 or peak flow.

Inhaled antibiotics from a nebuliser are advocated by some but have not been shown to be superior to intravenous regimens. A combination of gentamicin and carbenicillin (in sequence rather than as a mixture as they inactivate each other in solution), or colistin may be given twice daily. Attacks of wheezing may occur after the first doses of colistin.

Haemoptysis

This usually subsides with energetic treatment of infection. Vitamin K should be given if liver disease is present and has caused a coagulation defect.

Pneumothorax

A small pneumothorax causing little or no increase in breathlessness needs no active treatment. A larger pneumothorax will require tube drainage but recurrence is common and surgical treatment of repeated pneumothoraces is tolerated surprisingly well. Surgical treatment is necessary if tube drainage is not successful after a week.

Malabsorption

Many older patients can abandon regular pancreatic supplements without developing troublesome diarrhoea or weight loss. The fat intake should however probably be kept low.

Abdominal pain and intestinal obstruction

It is important to recognise 'meconium ileus equivalent', as surgical treatment of obstruction gives very poor results. The condition should be treated medically with intravenous fluids and administration of acetylcysteine as 10 ml of a 20% solution q.d.s. orally or through a naso-gastric tube, with 100 ml of a 10% solution q.d.s. as an enema.

Genetic counselling

Male patients will be infertile. Advice to female patients about the wisdom of pregnancy will be based on the possible harmful effects of pregnancy on the mother's health and on her ability to care for a child, as well as on genetic factors. All unaffected siblings of patients will be heterozygotes and must be warned about the risk of transmitting the disease should they marry another heterozygote. Sweat tests should be carried out on children of siblings. Unfortunately there is still no method of identifying heterozygotes other than by family history nor is there any certain method of intrauterine diagnosis. Advice to parents of children with cystic fibrosis can be based only on information about the likelihood of producing another affected child.

24. INHALED FOREIGN BODY

Inhalation of a foreign body into the bronchial tree occurs most often in children of toddler age. Older children and adults can usually describe an episode of choking in which 'something went down the wrong way' unless they have been under the influence of drugs or alcohol, have had a period of reduced consciousness, or suffer from a neurological disease affecting the swallowing mechanism. Chronic neurological disease rarely results in inhalation of a single foreign body and the clinical picture is therefore different.

Inhalation of a foreign body should be suspected if:

— Sudden collapse with cyanosis and loss of consciousness occurs while eating (the so called 'cafe-coronary')
— A bout of choking is followed by breathlessness, wheezing or persistent coughing
— Pneumonia or lung abscess follows a bout of choking by days, weeks or even months
— A child or susceptible adult develops lower lobe collapse, pneumonia or abscess.

History

— What happened? How likely is it that a foreign body was inhaled at that time?
— If the patient is a child, was the episode of choking witnessed?
— How long ago did it occur?
— What was, or might have been, inhaled? How big was it, what was it made of and what shape was it? If you are in doubt whether such material might be radio-opaque the patient or a parent may be able to give you a piece of similar material. The composition of a foreign body is important. A non radio-opaque boiled sweet, currant or peanut may cause severe local bronchial damage and, unless removed immediately, may result in later loss of a lobe or lung
— What symptoms, if any, have occurred since?

Examination of the chest

There may be no abnormal physical signs. This is because the foreign body may not, as yet, have blocked a bronchus, or because you cannot detect obstruction of a lobar or segmental bronchus on clinical examination. Breath sounds may be reduced on one side. This is more common children than adults. Wheeze may range from severe stridor, suggesting a foreign body in the larynx or trachea, to a quiet expiratory wheeze heard over one lung. Signs of lobar collapse with or without infection may occur later if the foreign body remains.

Chest X-ray

Within hours
> — May be normal, particularly if only inspiratory films are obtained. Expiratory films are essential if inhaled foreign bodies are not radio-opaque)
> — May show an opaque foreign body (most inhaled foreign bodies are not radio-opaque)
> — May show 'air trapping' in one lobe or lung. This is difficult or impossible to detect on the usual inspiratory films but expiratory films may reveal air trapping with increased translucency in the affected lung or lobe. (An expiratory film on a toddler can be obtained by making the child cry!). In the majority of children who have inhaled a foreign body the chest X-ray is abnormal but well-centred inspiratory and expiratory films are necessary to detect air trapping.

Within days
> — May still be normal or may show an opaque foreign body
> — May show collapse of a lobe or lung.

Within weeks
May show consolidation, collapse or abscess with or without the shadow of the inhaled foreign body.

Management

> 1. First-aid treatment of life-threatening inhaled foreign body (e.g. 'cafe-coronary'). 'Heimlich manoeuvre': stand behind the patient or kneel over a face-down recumbent patient; place your arms round his chest with a closed first over the xiphisternum and put your other hand over your fist. With a sharp jerking movement force your fist up under the xiphisternum. This may dislodge the foreign body
> 2. *Never disregard an adult's or older child's description of a choking episode in which 'something went down the wrong way' even if you find no abnormality on clinical examination or on the chest X-ray.* Failure to remove a foreign body early may lead to

loss of a lobe or a whole lung. The diagnosis can be excluded only by bronchoscopy.

If there are any abnormal clinical or X-ray changes do not be swayed by an optimistic parent's hope that the child probably coughed the foreign body out again

3. Do not delay bronchoscopy if the story of inhalation is convincing, if there are abnormal physical signs or if the X-ray is abnormal. Delay may make removal of a foreign body difficult or impossible.

   The rigid bronchoscope is far superior to the fibreoptic bronchoscope for removal of a foreign body. If there is real uncertainty as to whether an adult has inhaled a foreign body it is reasonable to perform a fibreoptic bronchoscopy if that is more easily arranged than a rigid bronchoscopy. It must be recognised however that, if a foreign body is seen, a rigid bronchoscopy may then be necessary to remove it.

   Attempts to remove foreign bodies require an experienced bronchoscopist. Removing material from the bronchial tree may be difficult and clumsy handling may result in fragmentation of friable material

4. If a single foreign body has been cleanly removed soon after inhalation further complications are unlikely. If the foreign body might have fragmented, if it had been in place for some time, or if it was an organic material likely to produce local inflammatory changes, further follow-up with chest X-ray for a few weeks is wise.

Later complications of inhaled foreign bodies are discussed in the chapters on pneumonia, lung abscess and bronchiectasis.

25. ACUTE THROMBO-EMBOLISM

Diagnosis

The possibility of pulmonary thrombo-embolism is all too often overlooked because the symptoms and signs may appear to be trivial and are not specific. In general, small pulmonary emboli may produce slight or no symptoms, moderate sized emboli if associated with pulmonary infarction cause respiratory symptoms, whilst large emboli cause 'cardiac' symptoms as a result of obstruction to much of the pulmonary circulation. *As no symptom or sign is specific to pulmonary thrombo-embolism it is important to consider the diagnosis whenever a patient at increased risk develops symptoms or signs, however slight, which are compatible with the diagnosis.*

The risk of thrombo-embolism is increased in people with one or more of the following risk factors:

— Previous pulmonary embolism
— Obese, bed-bound or immobile
— Varicose veins
— Malignant disease
— Taking the contraceptive pill
— Recent surgical treatment (particularly hip or pelvic surgery) or lower limb trauma
— Pregnancy or puerperium
— Atrial fibrillation or congestive heart failure
— Recent myocardial infarction
— Previous deep venous thrombosis.

Common symptoms

— Sudden breathlessness, which may be transient or may persist
— Chest pain, usually but not always pleuritic (may be anginal)
— Cough
— Haemoptysis, often small, repeated, pure blood
— Apprehension, sweating
— Syncope (suggests massive embolism)
— Worsening of existing right heart failure.

In general the larger the emboli the more severe the symptoms. There have often been similar but less troublesome symptoms for several days before the patient is first seen.

Common physical signs

There may be no abnormal signs or one or more of the following may be found:
— Rapid respiratory rate
— Rapid pulse (not invariable even after massive pulmonary embolism)
— Expiratory wheeze (from bronchoconstriction secondary to embolism)
— Pleural friction rib
— Fever
— Loud pulmonary component of second heart sound
— Hypotension (suggests massive embolism)
— Gallop rhythm and/or pulmonary systolic murmur
— Signs of consolidation or pleural effusion
— Evidence of deep venous thrombosis (not common at the time of pulmonary embolism).

Massive pulmonary embolism

This has occurred if the embolism is associated with severe haemodynamic disturbance and implies that more than 50% of the pulmonary arterial tree has been obstructed.

Symptoms and signs

The essence of the clinical picture is sudden breathlessness with right ventricular failure and shock – hence:
— Sudden severe breathlessness with rapid respiratory rate
— Elevated jugular venous pressure
— Low systolic blood pressure
— Cyanosis
— Cold, poorly perfused peripheries
— Gallop rhythm
— There may be no tachycardia and the pulmonary component of the second heart sound is often not loud. The patient often prefers to lie flat and may faint if sat up.

Investigation

Chest X-ray

There are no specific radiographic changes and the chest X-ray often shows no abnormality. After massive pulmonary embolism there may be oligaemic areas in the affected lobes.

Later non-specific changes include:-
— An area of consolidation, usually adjacent to the pleura and often basal
— Elevation of a diaphragm
— Pleural effusion, often small
— Linear shadows, unilateral or bilateral.

Electrocardiogram
This is not a sensitive investigation for pulmonary embolus, and is often normal. However it may show an S wave in Lead I and a Q wave with T wave inversion in lead III, right bundle branch block or right axis deviation. Large emboli are more likely than small to affect the ECG, which is abnormal in the great majority of patients after massive embolism.

Isotope lung scan (see Chapter 9)
This should be performed as soon as possible, ideally within 24 hours, because small pulmonary emboli resolve rapidly in previously fit patients and the lung scan may have reverted to normal if the investigation is delayed.

Pulmonary angiogram (see Chapter 6)
Usually clinicians are prepared to rely on clinical, radiographic and lung scan evidence when reaching a diagnosis and deciding treatment. Pulmonary angiography is required when the diagnosis is in doubt, when thrombolytic therapy or any form of surgical therapy is considered, or when there are special risks of anticoagulation.

Lower limb venography
This is of no diagnostic value in relation to pulmonary embolism. Venograms may be normal after pulmonary embolism either because the source of embolus was elsewhere or because no clot remains in the leg veins, or they may be abnormal in patients with conditions other than pulmonary embolism.

Arterial blood gases
Arterial gases may be normal after small emboli but after larger emboli hypoxia with slightly reduced Pa_{CO_2} is characteristic. Pa_{CO_2} may occasionally rise after massive pulmonary emboli.

Serum enzyme measurements
These are of little diagnostic value as serum lactic dehydrogenase (for example) is often normal after embolism and, if abnormal, does not help distinguish between embolism and other conditions such as pneumonia or congestive failure.

TREATMENT

Small and moderate sized pulmonary emboli

1. Anticoagulate with heparin in an initial single dose of 5000 units followed by a continuous intravenous infusion of 1000–1500 units hourly. For effective anticoagulation and lowest risk of bleeding heparin dosage should be adjusted according to results of serial coagulation test (the tests preferred vary between laboratories). Heparin acts only to prevent further venous thrombosis and hence prevent further embolism, and has no effect on existing emboli in the lung

2. Begin oral anticoagulation with warfarin 10 mg daily for 3 days. This takes 2–3 days to increase the prothrombin time, and subsequent dosage is guided by results of prothrombin time estimations. The duration of oral anticoagulation is controversial but it would seem reasonable to stop treatment after 3–6 months if a patient has had only one bout of embolism and if, after that period of treatment, no obvious predisposing factors are still present.

Massive pulmonary embolism

Treatment must start immediately.

1. Lie the patient flat and give oxygen at high concentration
2. Set up an intravenous infusion (and consider giving Dextran 70 0.5 litres if the patient is shocked)
3. Give I.V. heparin 10 000–15 000 units immediately (to counter the pulmonary vasconstriction associated with pulmonary embolism). Start infusion of heparin 25 units/kg per hour

Thrombolytic therapy

Unless there is rapid improvement thrombolytic therapy with streptokinase (or urokinase) should be considered (see below for contraindications).

For this treatment the collaboration of a radiologist (for angiography), a haematologist (for advice on drug dosage) and, we recommend, a cardiologist (for advice on treatment of dysrhythmias or circulatory support) are invaluable.

1. Arrange an immediate pulmonary angiogram to confirm the diagnosis
2. Insert a float catheter into the pulmonary artery to monitor cardiac output and pulmonary artery pressure and also to administer thrombolytic therapy directly into the pulmonary arteries
3. Assess the coagulation status of the patient (especially if, as is common, anticoagulants have already been given), and plan subsequent coagulation tests for control of streptokinase dosage

4. Give a loading dose of 250 000–600 000 units of streptokinase over 30 minutes together with 100 mg hydrocortisone hemisuccinate to reduce the risk of hypersensitivity reaction
5. Continue with a maintenance dose of 100 000 units hourly, the dosage being adjusted according to results of repeated coagulation tests. If emboli are lysed blood pressure, peripheral perfusion, pulse and respiratory rate should improve and measurements will show an increase of cardiac output and a fall of pulmonary artery pressure
6. If improvement occurs thrombolytic therapy can be stopped after 24–48 hours, to be followed by heparin, and subsequently warfarin anticoagulation.

Streptokinase is contraindicated in patients who have had recent major surgery, are known to have a risk of bleeding from peptic ulcer, who have severe liver disease, previous cerebrovascular accident, severe hypertension or who are pregnant or post-partum.

Complications and risks of thrombolytic therapy. Haemorrhage is the major risk but febrile reactions or anaphylaxis may occur. There may be profuse bleeding from recent sites of venepuncture, arterial puncture or cut-down sites. If this is severe thrombolytic action can be halted by I.V. infusion of 10–20 ml of 10% epsilon aminocaproic acid each hour.

Surgical embolectomy
Failure of thrombolytic therapy may necessitate surgical embolectomy for which transfer to a specialised unit is essential as cardio-pulmonary bypass is required.

Later course

Nearly all patients with pulmonary embolism show complete clinical and haemodynamic recovery and complete or almost complete radiological and angiographic resolution within 4–6 weeks. Chronic pulmonary hypertension and cor pulmonale rarely follow acute pulmonary embolism.

Further pulonary emboli can usually be prevented by anticoagulation but if this fails or is contraindicated and if emboli are believed to have originated from the legs or abdomen surgical interruption of the inferior vena cava may be advised.

26. PNEUMOTHORAX

Air may enter the pleural cavity:
1. from the lung – in a patient with apparently healthy lungs or with previous lung disease such as emphysema, asthma, cystic fibrosis, pulmonary fibrosis or staphylococcal pneumonia
2. through the chest wall after chest trauma or medical procedures such as pleural aspiration or insertion of a CVP line
3. through the diaphragm after trauma (rare)
4. from gas-forming organisms in the pleural cavity (rare).

Suspect a pneumothorax in a patient with:
1. sudden pleuritic chest pain often, but not always, with breathlessness, and sometimes with a single small haemoptysis
2. rapid development of breathlessness without chest pain
3. reduced movement of one side of the chest
4. reduced breath sounds with normal, or increased, resonance to percussion ('resonance with silence').

Note: the trachea remains in the midline unless 'tension' has developed.

Suspicion of a pneumothorax is increased:
— in tall thin young men – apical bullae without other lung disease are common in this group
— with pre-existing lung disease (emphysema, asthma, fibrotic lung disease, cystic fibrosis, staphylococcal pneumonia)
— after recent chest trauma, chest aspiration, lung biopsy or insertion of a CVP line.

Confirmation of pneumothorax

Unless the patient is severely breathless with an obvious pneumothorax a chest X-ray is essential. Look for the line of the visceral pleura in the upper chest and the lack of blood vessels beyond it. A small pneumothorax is better seen on an expiratory film. A decubitus film is valuable if the patient cannot sit up. Beware of confusing a large emphysematous bulla with a pneumothorax. Occasionally a pneumothorax is associated with sufficient bleeding into the pleural cavity for a fluid level to be present (haemopneumothorax).

128

Differential diagnosis
1. Pleuritic pain from any other cause
2. Pulmonary embolus may cause similar symptoms of pain, breathlessness and haemoptysis
3. Emphysematous bullae may cause similar physical signs to pneumothorax.

MANAGEMENT

Not all patients with pneumothorax require removal of air. Air in the pleural cavity is slowly absorbed and no specific treatment is needed if:
— the patient is young and is not breathless
— there is no evidence of lung disease as judged by either previous symptoms or the chest X-ray
— there is less than 3 cm of air around the lung on the chest X-ray
— the respiratory rate is less than 20 per min
— the pulse rate is less than 100/min.
If after a short period of observation the patient is still not breathless there is no need for treatment in hospital. Advise the patient against vigorous exercise, flying or underwater diving, and to report immediately to the hospital if symptoms recur or increase. If, for any reason, it is decided to remove air from such a patient's pneumothorax simple aspiration (see below) will suffice.

Removal of air

The lung will usually expand rapidly if the air in the pleural space is removed. An intercostal tube should be inserted in any of the following circumstances:
— The patient is breathless at rest
— The pneumothorax is large (more than about 3 cm between the edge of the lung and the chest wall on chest X-ray)
— There is evidence of continued air leak:
  a. Increasing breathlessness
  b. Rising pulse and/or respiratory rate
  c. Enlarging pneumothorax on serial chest X-rays
— There is 'tension' as shown by:
  a. Deviation of the trachea away from the side of the pneumothorax
  b. Displacement of the mediastinum away from the side of the pneumothorax (judged by position of apex beat or, better, by chest X-ray)
  c. Falling blood pressure, rapid pulse and respiratory rate, sweating and distress

— There is subcutaneous emphysema which is more than slight
or which is increasing
— There is underlying lung disease especially:
a. With stiff lungs which may re-expand only with difficulty
b. Emphysema or asthma
c. If previous symptoms suggest obstruction of the bronchus
in the collapsed lung (as by carcinoma) which will prevent
re-aeration
— There is more than a small amount of fluid in the pleura –
which is presumably blood.

Technique of removing air

In an emergency
If a patient with a definite or strongly suspected pneumothorax is severely
breathless, pale, sweating, hypotensive or has a marked tachycardia air
must be removed as a matter of urgency. Any available needle or
cannula can be inserted into the second intercostal space anteriorly in the
mid-clavicular line or the 4th or 5th space in the axilla. Air will be heard
to escape with a hiss. This emergency treatment should, of course, be
followed as soon as possible by insertion of a chest tube.

Simple aspiration
A large size Teflon intravenous cannula is inserted between the ribs in
either of the sites described in the next section and air is gently aspirated
with a 60 ml syringe and a 3-way tap and is expelled under water.
Aspiration is stopped when resistance is felt (if about 4 litres has been
removed and no resistance is felt it is usually found that no expansion has
occurred in which case air must still be leaking from the lung and an
intercostal tube is required for continued drainage). When resistance is
felt and no more air can be removed the cannula can be removed.

Intercostal tube drainage
The technique of insertion of an intercostal tube is described in Chapter
41.

Preferred sites
Either the 4th or 5th intercostal space in the anterior or mid-axillary line
(this site is less likely than an anterior site to leave an unsightly scar); or
the 2nd. intercostal space anteriorly in the mid-clavicular line (lateral to the
internal mammary artery).

Choice of tube
Our preference is for the Argyll, or similar, thoracic catheter attached
either to an underwater seal or to a flutter valve. *It is important that the safe
method of introducing the tube described in Chapter 41 is used.*

Underwater seal
The purpose of the underwater seal is:
1. to permit air to escape from, but not to re-enter, the tube

2. to show that the tube is not blocked and is in the pleural
   space – initially by noting bubbling of air, later by noting
   oscillation of the column of water with respiration, which
   rises up the tube during inspiration
3. to show continued removal of air by noting bubbling.

*Note: It is important that the end of the tube is not more than 2–3 cm below
the surface of the water. A greater depth offers a significant resistance to the
escape of air.*

The flutter valve ('Heimlich valve')

This is a light-weight disposable one-way valve which can be attached to
the end of the intercostal tube. (*Note: ensure that the valve is fitted in the
correct direction to allow, and not prevent, escape of air!*). It is as effective as
an underwater seal for removal of air.

Advantages of flutter valve over underwater seal:
   — The patient is free to move around as he wishes and is not
     'tied' to a long tube and a bottle
   — Moving the patient to an X-ray department or to another
     hospital is easier and safer.

Disadvantages of flutter valve:
   — It is difficult to detect occasional or slow escape of air.
   — It is not of use for confirming that the tube is within the
     pleural cavity
   However for both these purposes the distal end of the flutter
   valve can be connected temporarily by tubing to an underwater
   seal
   — Most importantly, the valve may become blocked if fluid
     enters it and a flutter valve is therefore not suitable if there is
     more than a trace of pleural fluid.

As air is removed the lung re-expands and the flow of air usually
ceases within 24 hours. When there is no further flow of air from the
tube, even on coughing:
   1. Observe the underwater seal
      If the column of water oscillates with breathing then the tube
      is in the pleural space and the lung is probably expanded. If
      the column of water does not oscillate then the lung may
      have expanded and occluded the end of the tube or the tube
      may have become blocked or kinked but the pneumothorax
      persists.
   2. Arrange PA chest X-ray in expiration to confirm if the lung is
      fully, or almost fully, expanded
   3. Clamp the tube for 24 hours. If during this time the patient
      becomes breathless release the clamp and observe if air
      bubbles from the tube
   4. Repeat the expiration chest X-ray
   5. If there is little or no residual pneumothorax remove the
      tube.

Note: *It is pointless and is potentially dangerous to clamp a chest tube for more than a few moments while air is flowing from it, for inevitably the air will then accumulate in the pleural space. The tube and valve system must remain unobstructed while the patient is moved or while any other procedures are being carried out.*

Some problems in management of pneumothorax

Bubbling of air persists for more than 24 hours
This indicates a persisting leak of air from either:
1. the lung from the initial tear or, all too often, from insertion of the tube into the lung due to to faulty or careless technique of insertion
2. From outside the chest through the chest wall and into the pleural space

Prevention
1. Ensure an airtight seal around the tube if the second cause is suspected
2. Apply suction (large volume, low vacuum) to the bottle or valve in an attempt to remove air faster than it can leak from the lung
3. If a small intercostal tube had been used, it may be necessary to replace it with a larger one to allow larger volumes of air to be removed.

Note: *Low-volume, high-vacuum suction is ineffective and potentially dangerous as it limits the volume of air which can be removed and may pull the lung onto the end of the tube hence preventing further flow of air.*

Once section has been started it should continue without interruption until the lung has re-expanded and has remained so for 24 hours.

The lung still does not re-expand
If this occurs and air flow persists either during suction or whenever suction is removed, consult a thoracic surgeon. It may be necessary to:
1. Insert a second intercostal tube to increase the volume of air removed. The two tubes must be connected via a 'Y' connector to the same underwater seal to which suction is applied. If attached to separate underwater seals unequal suction on the two bottles may cause water to be drawn from one bottle into the chest
2. Advise surgical pleurectomy or pleurodesis. Even patients with severe underlying lung disease may be at less risk from early surgical treatment than from prolonged intubation.

If a patient is considered unfit for surgical treatment an attempt may be made to produce chemical pleurodesis by introducing 500 mg tetracycline into the pleural space diluted in 50 ml saline, or introducing talc at thoracoscopy.

The patient becomes distressed as air is removed from the pleural space

1. If air is removed too fast pulmonary oedema may develop. Allow some air to re-enter the pleural space by momentarily disconnecting the intercostal tube from the underwater seal, and then remove air more slowly.
   Oxygen therapy and intravenous diuretics may be required

2. If the bronchus to the collapsed lung has become occluded by secretions (or if it contains a tumour) air cannot re-enter the lung as the pneumothorax is drained and the mediastinum is rapidly pulled to the side of the pneumothorax. Disconnect the intercostal tube from the underwater seal to allow air to re-enter the pleural space. Bronchoscopy is then required to establish the cause of the bronchial obstruction and if possible remove it.

Surgical treatment by pleurectomy or pleurodesis

These methods are usually required:
   — if an air leak persists or if the lung fails to expand after suction through a correctly positioned tube
   — after two or three pneumothoraces on one side or after bilateral pneumothoraces
   — If the patient is an underwater diver or an aircraft pilot or crew member.

27. PLEURAL EFFUSION

A pleural effusion should be suspected in a patient with:
- — Progressive shortness of breath on exertion, expecially if preceded by pleuritic pain
- — Dullness to percussion at one or both bases associated with diminished breath sounds
- — A chest X-ray showing a basal homogenous opacity with a curvilinear meniscus at its upper lateral aspect.

Note that:
- — Loculated effusions may lead to a variety of other appearances
- — Fluid levels are seen only if there is air as well as liquid in the pleural space, i.e. a hydro- or haemo-pneumothorax
- — An effusion may not be apparent if only a supine chest X-ray is available or may cause general opacification of the affected hemithorax. If there is doubt whether a pleural effusion is present and for any reason an erect film cannot be taken, a decubitus film will show the fluid running away from the base of the lung by gravity. Ultrasound is a useful method of confirming and localising pleural fluid. A diagnostic tap may be required to be certain of the presence of fluid.

DIAGNOSIS OF THE CAUSE OF AN EFFUSION

Clinical clues

- — *Bilateral pleural effusion* suggests heart failure (other Ɪ features will be apparent), hypoproteinaemia (oedema and ascites common), widespread malignancy, pulmonary emboli or connective tissue disease
- — *If the patient is a previously healthy young adult* consider tuberculosis. A tuberculous pleural effusion may or may not be associated with pain, fever or systemic symptoms

— *Is there chest pain?*
   Pleuritic pain, consider:
   a. Pneumonia – has there been any recent febrile illness or
      productive cough?
   b. Pulmonary embolism – look for evidence of peripheral
      venous thrombosis and seek any predisposing causes (see
      Chapter 25)
   c. Connective tissue disorder – SLE (any systemic illness or
      arthralgia?), rheumatoid disease – (any arthritis?)
   Non-pleuritic pain, consider:
   a. Cardiac pain – any evidence of recent myocardial
      infarction with resulting heart failure or post-infarction
      syndrome (of which pleuritic pain may be a feature)
   b. Non-cardiac pain – aortic dissection which can lead to
      haemothorax; oesophageal perforation (any dysphagia?),
      tumour of chest wall, bronchial carcinoma or pleural
      mesothelioma (any palpable mass or localised tenderness
      of the chest wall?)
— *Is there fever?*
   Fever may be due to either the underlying cause of the effusion
   (e.g. pneumonia, sub-phrenic abscess) or may indicate that the
   pleural fluid itself is infected (empyema)
— *Has there been loss of weight?* This suggests malignancy,
   tuberculosis or chronic empyema
— *Is there evidence of heart disease* such as orthopnoea, signs
   of left or right heart failure, pulsus paradoxus or cardiac
   murmur?
— *Are there abdominal symptoms or signs?* Pain (pancreatitis
   may cause left-sided pleural effusions); ascites is frequently
   accompanied by pleural effusion; recent abdominal surgery
   or intestinal perforation (subphrenic abscess); vomiting
   (ruptured oesophagus); enlarged liver and/or spleen
   (cirrhosis, lymphoma)
— *Is there any reason for hypoproteinaemia* (malnutrition,
   malabsorption, nephrotic syndrome, cirrhosis)?
— *Are there joint symptoms?* Rheumatoid arthritis may cause
   painless pleural effusions; several connective tissue disorders
   may cause arthralgia
— *Is there evidence of malignancy?* Consider specially
   bronchial carcinoma, breast carcinoma, renal carcinoma or
   pleural mesothelioma. Rapid recurrence of blood stained or
   clear pleural effusions after aspiration suggests malignancy
— *Is there a history of recent trauma* to the chest wall or
   possibly to the thoracic duct?
— *Has there been occupational exposure to asbestos?* (Benign
   effusion or mesothelioma).

Radiological clues

Only effusions of more than 300 ml are visible on standard chest
X-rays; smaller effusions may be seen on decubitus views.

— Bilateral pleural effusion (see 'clinical clues')
— A large effusion without displacement of the mediastinum
  implies collapse of the underlying lung which is usually due to
  a carcinoma obstructing the bronchus
— Tumour mass visible in the lung suggests malignancy
— Consolidation due to pneumonia seen in addition to the
  effusion
— Lymphangitis or enlarged lymph nodes suggest malignancy
— Erosion or destruction of ribs suggests malignancy
— Enlarged heart suggests heart disease or pericardial effusion.

PLEURAL ASPIRATION

The nature of an effusion cannot be determined from the chest X-ray,
therefore all pleural effusions should be aspirated unless:

— left ventricular failure, ascites or hypoalbuminaemia are
  present in which case the response to treatment may be
  sufficient confirmation of the cause of the effusion
— the effusion is very small or is improving spontaneously
— the effusion is known to be of long-standing and not to be
  increasing
— knowledge of the cause of an effusion would not influence
  management.

Technique of diagnostic aspiration

The best site for aspiration is judged from both clinical examination and
from inspection of the X-ray. If, as is usual, the fluid is free (i.e. not
loculated) the patient sits, with the arms crossed and resting comfortably
on a support in front of him. By percussion the upper level of dullness is
identified and a site chosen just below this level and medial to the
scapula. A common error is to insert the needle too low when attempting
to sample a small effusion. The diaphragm may well be raised in such a
patient and the needle will then pass through or below the diaphragm.

   Having explained the procedure to the patient the skin is cleaned and
local anaesthetic (2% lignocaine is adequate) is injected first into the skin
and then generously into the chest wall. As the needle is advanced the
plunger is repeatedly withdrawn until pleural fluid enters the syringe. The
needle is then removed and a diagnostic specimen aspirated into a 20 or
50 ml syringe.

If the effusion is localised or loculated the site for aspiration is judged by careful measurement on the X-ray or by ultrasound. Always note in the records the site of diagnostic aspiration and the appearance, and smell if any, of the fluid removed.

Examination of pleural fluid

Before a diagnostic aspiration consider which investigations will be required on the fluid.

Microscopic

Collect at least 10 ml of fluid for microscopic examination. Polymorph neutrophils suggest bacterial inflammation and if present in large numbers suggest a developing empyema. A predominantly lymphocytic effusion is typical of tuberculosis but is common in a chronic effusion of any cause. Excessive eosinophils usually reflect bleeding into the fluid but may be present in larger numbers (over 20% of the total white cells) when the patients has a blood eosinophilia of any cause or rarely in malignant effusions or those due to connective tissue diseases.

Fluid should be examined for malignant cells only if malignancy is considered likely. This time consuming and technically demanding investigation should not be considered a routine for all undiagnosed pleural effusions. Failure to detect malignant cells does not exclude a malignant cause and false positive reports are not uncommon particularly from effusions due to infarction or infection. Pleural biopsy is a more satisfactory method of diagnosing pleural malignancy.

Microbiological

Pleural fluid collected for diagnosis should always be examined for bacteria. 10–20 ml of fluid collected into a sterile container should be sent immediately to the laboratory. Many laboratories do not examine specimens for tubercle bacilli unless specifically requested. If tuberculosis is seriously considered a large volume of fluid should be sent for examination (but pleural biopsy is a more satisfactory method of diagnosis). If the fluid is opaque, purulent or foul smelling then 10–20 ml should be collected in a sterile syringe, the air expelled and the syringe capped for immediate culture for anaerobic organisms.

Chemical

Protein estimation distinguishes exudates from transudates (see below). Glucose is estimated on a sample collected into a fluoride tube. Blood glucose should be measured at the same time. Glucose concentrations are often low in bacterial infection, malignancy and rheumatoid arthritis.

Amylase concentrations are much higher in pleural fluid than in serum when an effusion complicates acute pancreatitis or perforation of the oesophagus.

The nature of the pleural fluid

It is important to note the appearance and smell of the material which is aspirated. A foul smell suggests anaerobic infection.

Transudate

The fluid will have a protein content less than 30 grams/litre. Transudates are often bilateral and may be due to:

— *raised pulmonary venous pressure*: left ventricular failure (common); mitral stenosis (uncommon); constrictive pericarditis (rare)

— *hypoalbuminaemia*: malnutrition, malabsorption, nephrotic syndrome, cirrhosis

— *fibrosing mediastinitis or myxoedema* (very rare).

Exudate

If the fluid protein content is more than 30 grams/litre, this may be due to:

— *inflammation*: pneumonia, subphrenic abscess, pulmonary infarction, connective tissue disorders, pancreatitis, post-myocardial infarction syndrome

— *neoplasms involving the pleura*: malignant effusions are often blood stained and recur rapidly after aspiration; primary pleural mesothelioma; secondary carcinoma (commonly breast, bronchus, kidney); lymphoma

— *disorders of lymph drainage*: (yellow nails syndrome, suggested by lymphoedema of limbs and yellow discolouration of the nails).

Pus (empyema)

This most often occurs during or after pneumonia, when the organism is that of the pneumonia (often *Strep. pneumoniae* or *Staph. pyogenes*). In the absence of obvious preceding pneumonia the infection is often mixed containing anaerobes, microaerophilic organisms and gram-negative and positive bacteria. Tuberculosis, actinomycosis or amoebiasis may also cause empyemas. Empyema may complicate sub-phrenic, hepatic or perinephric abscess, bronchiectasis, ruptured oesophagus or chest trauma, including penetrating chest wounds and thoracic surgery.

Blood

Blood from haemorrhage defibrinates leaves an effusion together with a thick fibrin deposit on the surfaces of the pleura. The commonest causes are trauma, anticoagulant therapy or dissecting or leaking aortic aneurysm, but haemothorax may occasionally accompany spontaneous pneumothorax. Blood staining is most commonly due to malignancy or pulmonary infarction, but may be seen after pneumonia or in tuberculous effusions.

Chylous and pseudochylous effusions

These are opaque and appear milky and must be distinguished from empyema. On standing chylous effusions develop a creamy top layer in contrast to empyema fluid from which pus sediments to the bottom. Chemical analysis of chylous effusions show large amounts of triglycerides and some cholesterol, and chylomicra are visible under the microscope as fat globules which stain with Sudan III.

Chylous effusions follow obstruction or leakage of the thoracic duct usually due to chest trauma or intrathoracic lymphoma.

Pseudochylous effusion contains large numbers of cholesterol crystals which can be seen under a microscope, but do not stain with Sudan III, and may accumulate in chronic pleural effusions of any cause.

Ascitic fluid

This may cross the diaphragm to enter the pleural cavity, almost always on the right, whatever the cause of the ascites. Pleural effusion may also develop in patients undergoing peritoneal dialysis. Depending on the cause of the ascites it may have features of a transudate or exudate or may be blood stained. It cannot be differentiated from primary pleural fluid unless the presence and significance of the ascites is recognised.

Gut contents

Perforation or rupture of the oesophagus.

Pleural biopsy (see Chapter 12)

A pleural biopsy should be performed in every patient at the time of initial diagnostic aspiration unless the fluid is purulent. The reasons for recommending biopsy at this stage are:
— Biopsy is more likely to yield a diagnosis of malignancy or tuberculosis than examination of pleural fluid
— Biopsy is unlikely to yield false positive reports of malignancy, enables the cell type to be identified and is more satisfactory for diagnosis of lymphoma
— The opportunity for biopsy may be lost if an effusion resolves after diagnostic aspiration or if too little fluid remains for safe biopsy.

Thoracoscopy

Inspection of the pleural space and surfaces by passing a thoracoscope through the chest wall under general anaesthesia enables a large part of the pleura to be examined and biopsies to be taken under direct vision. It is of value:
— if a diagnosis has not been obtained after repeated pleural biopsy and a local pleural cause for the effusion is suspected
— if lymphoma is suspected as a cause of effusion and no abnormality is found elsewhere. Characterisation of lymphoma requires larger biopsies than can usually be obtained by needle biopsy.

Thoracotomy

This is occasionally required to establish the cause of a persisting or recurring pleural effusion. The advent of thoracoscopy has reduced the need for thoracotomy.

Other investigations

- *Is the effusion tuberculous?* Pleural biopsy is the best method of diagnosis. It is wise also to examine sputum by smear and culture for tubercle bacilli and a tuberculin test should be performed on young people with an otherwise unexplained pleural effusion unless the diagnosis of tuberculosis has been established by pleural biopsy. It is uncommon to be able to see tubercle bacilli in the fluid of a tuberculous effusion and even culture may be negative
- *Is there a connective tissue disease?* Tests for antinuclear factor and rheumatoid factor in the blood may be of diagnostic value. Rheumatoid factor may be present in pleural fluid in other conditions and its presence does not therefore confirm that the effusion is due to rheumatoid disease
- *Is pulmonary infarction the cause?* Consider V/Q scan (see chapter 9) to seek defects in perfusion other than in the region of the effusion, but by the time an effusion is present such defects are rarely found
- *Is the effusion malignant?* Diagnosis rests on pleural biopsy or the finding of malignant cells in fluid. A search for the primary tumour is useful only if this will influence treatment. Specific treatment is, for example, available for small cell lung cancer, cancer of breast or prostate and for lymphoma
- *Is there a cardiac cause?* Echocardiography may show a valvular defect, poor left ventricular function or a pericardial effusion.

TREATMENT OF PLEURAL EFFUSION

1. No treatment may be needed if the effusion is asymptomatic and the underlying cause requires no treatment
2. Treat the underlying disease e.g. left ventricular failure
3. Pleural aspiration – a single aspiration may be sufficient if the effusion is small and does not recur e.g. post-pneumonic effusion
4. If a large effusion is to be drained it is preferable to insert a chest tube (see Chapter 41) through which fluid may be removed slowly and completely. It is unwise to remove more

than about 500 ml of fluid at a time. The tube can then be clamped for a few hours before another 500 ml is removed. Faster drainage of fluid may cause distress to the patients and can result in pulmonary oedema

5. Chemical pleurodesis is intended to obliterate the pleural space and hence prevent reaccumulation of fluid. It is considered only if an effusion is likely to recur and if no other treatment is available, usually therefore for malignant effusions and occasionally for those due to rheumatoid arthritis. It is essential to remove all the fluid, usually through an intercostal tube, before instilling the pleurodetic agent. Tetracycline 500 mg in 50 ml normal saline is our drug of choice but mepacrine, bleomycin or cyclophosphamide are alternatives. Whether the latter act by antitumour effects or as sclerosing agents is unknown. After instilling the drug the patient is positioned on his left, then right, side, front and back, standing and head down for 10 minutes in each position in an attempt to coat the whole pleural surface with the drug. The tube is left in place for a further 24 hours and then any fluid in the pleural space is drained before the tube is removed

6. Surgical treatment may be required for:
    a. Haemothorax, especially after trauma (see Chapter 34)
    b. Empyema (see below)
    c. Pleurectomy – this is rarely necessary after uncomplicated pleural effusions but is occasionally considered if a malignant effusion recurs despite chemical pleurodesis and the prognosis is otherwise good or after empyema or untreated haemothorax
    d. Ligation of thoracic duct for treatment of traumatic chylous effusions.

MANAGEMENT OF EMPYEMA

Management of an empyema is guided by the answers to the following questions.

1. What is the likely cause of the empyema?
    a. *Recent pneumonia* is the commonest (see Chapter 18). Empyema usually reflects ignored, delayed or inadequate antibiotic treatment of pneumonia but an underlying condition such as alcoholism, diabetes, rheumatoid arthritis, drug addiction, steroid therapy or immune deficiency should be considered. Empyema may develop as a sequel to infections beyond a bronchial carcinoma. Such underlying conditions may require treatment either together with, or soon after, treatment of the empyema

b. *Subdiaphragmatic infection* (subphrenic, hepatic or perinephric abscess) usually cause a serous pleural effusion but the abdominal organism may transgress the diaphragm to cause empyema. Treatment is required for the abdominal abscess as well as the empyema

c. *Recent aspiration of a pleural effusion* may have introduced infection. Fever following aspiration of pleural fluid should always suggest empyema.

d. Any history or evidence of *previous tuberculosis* in the thorax or elsewhere? Tuberculous empyema may develop many years after tuberculosis which became quiescent before the days of modern antituberculous therapy. Consider tuberculous empyema especially in patients who had pleural or chest wall procedures such as artificial pneumothoraces, plombage or thoracoplasty or who have extensive residual pleural shadowing

2. Is the empyema acute or chronic? It may be difficult to date the onset of symptoms due to empyema but an attempt to do so may be a guide to initial treatment. Radiologically loss of volume of a hemithorax with crowding of ribs indicates chronicity. The longer an empyema has been present the more likely it is that prolonged tube drainage or surgical decortication will be required

3. What is the infecting organism? Many acute empyemas contain anaerobic organisms and will be considered 'sterile' unless anaerobic cultures are requested. Likewise tuberculous empyema will be recognised only if appropriate staining and culture methods are used. Many other organisms may cause empyema. Their recognition will guide systemic or local chemotherapy but the principal method of treatment, whatever the organisms, is drainage of the fluid

4. What method of drainage is to be used? Pleural drainage is essential for all empyemas whatever the cause, character or infecting organism of the fluid. Systemic antibiotics are usually given also for acute empyemas.

a. *Simple aspiration*, usually repeatedly, through a wide-bore needle may sometimes suffice to remove most of the fluid from an acute empyema especially if the fluid is thin. Each aspiration is followed by instillation of an appropriate antibiotic into the pleural space before removing the needle. If the organism has not been identified benzyl penicillin in high dosage is probably the best systemic antibiotic in this situation. If repeated aspiration does not result in cure the fluid frequently becomes loculated into several separate collections. Drainage of each loculus may be very difficult and surgical treatment may then be

necessary. We find ultrasound helpful to identify the best
site for attempts to aspirate loculated pus

b. *Closed drainage* through an intercostal tube is usually
more successful than simple aspiration and is essential if
the pus is thick or has been present for several weeks. A
large lumen tube is essential to allow thick pus to drain
and to avoid blockage. A common and potentially
dangerous error is to insert the tube too low (see Chapter
41). Remember that the diaphragm is likely to be raised
below an empyema. Ultrasound is useful to identify the
exact site of a localised empyema as a guide to inserting a
drain. If closed drainage to an underwater seal (without
suction) is successful the fever will fall and the X-ray
improve. If the empyema becomes 'walled off' from the
rest of the pleural space (as judged by X-ray appearances)
serial instillation of radiological contrast medium (oily
propyliodone) through the tube allows the size and extent
of the empyema cavity to be defined. As the cavity
becomes smaller the tube is gradually withdrawn until no
empyema cavity remains, when the tube is removed.
Irrigation of localised empyema cavities through a double-
lumen tube with either noxythiolin 1% or an appropriate
antibiotic has recently been claimed to speed healing of
empyema

c. *Open drainage* involves resection of a small length of rib
and of chest wall to form a 'window' in the chest wall
through which pus can drain over a long period. This
method is an alternative to prolonged closed drainage of a
chronic empyema if decortication is not appropriate, and
has the advantage that the patient need not stay in
hospital during treatment

d. *Decortication* is required for some chronic empyemas and
for those which fail to respond to tube drainage.
Prolonged tube drainage can result in a long debilitating
period in hospital and we strongly recommend early
consultation with a thoracic surgeon when considering the
management of any patient with an empyema.

SPIRATORY PROBLEMS DUE TO CHEST WALL AND NEUROLOGICAL DISEASES

These conditions characteristically cause ventilatory failure and abnormal patterns of breathing without any pulmonary disease necessarily being present. Ventilatory failure initially occurs during sleep when the voluntary respiratory control system is relatively inactive and any abnormalities of the automatic control system are unmasked. Chest wall deformities and obesity add a restrictive load which the respiratory muscles have to cope with and which they, or the respiratory drive, may not be sufficient to overcome.

HYPOVENTILATION

Ventilatory failure should be suspected in the following situations.

The patient has a condition predisposing to hypoventilation

— *Chest wall disease.* The most important gross chest wall deformity is scoliosis but obesity can cause similar problems. Pectus excavatum, although often severe has little physiological effect and kyphosis and ankylosing spondylitis are also remarkably well tolerated

— *Diseases of peripheral nerves or respiratory muscles* such as infective polyneuritis, myasthenia gravis, poliomyelitis, dystrophia myotonica, muscular dystrophies, motor neurone disease. These may lead to respiratory failure in the presence of normal respiratory drive and chest shape because of the muscular weakness. If the diaphragm is paralysed bilaterally severe orthopnoea occurs and respiratory failure may develop at night

— *Disease of the respiratory centres.* Respiratory centres themselves may be damaged by multiple sclerosis, syringobulbia, brain stem infarction, tumours or poliomyelitis. Surgery in the posterior fossa of the skull and cervical cordotomy for intractable pain may also interrupt automatic respiratory pathways. In addition an idiopathic form of respiratory centre failure (central hypoventilation) occurs, mild forms of which are aggravated by any restrictive load on the chest (such as obesity).

Obstruction of the upper airways associated with obesity
In these circumstances there are symptoms, which are mainly
non-respiratory, to suggest hypoventilation:
- — snoring and snorting during sleep
- — frequent nightmares or waking at night breathless or
  distressed
- — early morning headaches (due to carbon dioxide retention)
- — sleepiness during the day
- — personality change
- — decrease in libido
- — frequent road traffic accidents due to daytime sleepiness.

There may be no complaint of breathlessness on exertion but respiratory
failure may be precipitated by an acute chest infection or by the addition
of mild airflow obstruction.

Physical signs are often unhelpful, but an attempt should be made to
watch the patient's breathing during sleep if possible. Other important
physical signs may be central cyanosis, somnolence and hypertension
which is a common association of chronic hypoxaemia.

Investigation

The possibility of hypoventilation should be investigated further in any
patient with one of the predisposing conditions who develops any of the
symptoms described above. This type of hypoventilation initially occurs
during sleep (or during acute intercurrent illness especially chest
infection), and therefore investigation during sleep is more useful than
measurements when awake.

Arterial blood gas analysis
The diagnosis rests on demonstrating hypercapnia with no primary
pulmonary or cardiac cause. Blood can be collected by arterial puncture
but sampling is then intermittent and the act of sampling often stimulates
respiration. An indwelling arterial line avoids this problem but sampling
is still intermittent and the technique is invasive. Non-invasive continuous
measurements with an ear oximeter (measuring oxygen saturation), or
with transcutaneous Po_2 and Pco_2 probes, depend on warming the skin
and arterialising the blood. The results agree well with arterial blood
analysis and continuous records can be obtained. Analysis during sleep is
essential to prove the diagnosis but hypoxaemia and hypercapnia are also
present by day in severe cases.

ECG
ECG monitoring of the patient during sleep will often detect
dysrhythmias, usually bradycardias, which are a frequent cause of death
in these patients.

Measurement of respiratory movements
If carried out with a magnetotometer or an impedance or inductance
spirometer these will confirm episodic hypoventilation as will
measurement of gas flow at the nose using a thermistor.

Note: Measurement of vital capacity or of other indicators of the function of the *voluntary* respiratory pathways are of limited use in assessing nocturnal hypoventilation, but serial measurements of vital capacity are essential in diseases of peripheral nerves or muscle (such as infective polyneuritis, poliomyelitis or myasthenia gravis) in which ventilatory function may deteriorate rapidly.

Haemoglobin
Polycythaemia may develop in response to chronic hypoxaemia.

Assessment
Assessment of pulmonary hypertension is by ECG, echo-cardiogram or right heart catheterisation. Alveolar hypoxia causes pulmonary arteriolar constriction and consequent pulmonary hypertension.

Treatment of sleep hypoventilation

1. Never give oxygen without measuring the blood gases before and during treatment. 24% is usually the most which can be tolerated by such patients without a dangerous rise in P_{CO_2}. Oxygen therapy which is safe while the patient is awake may be fatal when he falls asleep and repeated blood gas measurements, ideally by a non-invasive method, are therefore necessary for safety
2. Never give any sedation (e.g. hypnotics or antidepressants). Even alcohol may cause dangerous depression of ventilation
3. If the patient is obese a drastic diet is indicated
4. Airflow obstruction from asthma, chronic bronchitis or acute bronchitis must be treated energetically
5. Respiratory stimulant drugs. Intravenous doxapram is useful in an acute situation but there are no satisfactory long-term respiratory stimulants, although medroxyprogestrone, dichlorphenamide and almitrine have all been used
6. Mechanical ventilation. Positive pressure ventilation may be carried out through an endotracheal tube but it is usually very difficult to wean such patients off this type of ventilation. A tracheostomy is therefore often necessary and this may be difficult to close, or may lead to tracheal stenosis with an unwelcome increase in resistance to air flow. If the larynx is competent external negative pressure ventilation is therefore preferable but expertise in this technique is found only in special centres. A cuirass, a Tunnicliffe jacket or a tank respirator (iron lung) are all effective. The iron lung is inconvenient for long-term use but the other methods can be used for long-term assisted ventilation in the patient's home, particularly as it is often required only at night
7. Tracheostomy may be necessary for intermittent positive pressure ventilation in an emergency situation but is best

avoided because of problems of delayed closure or of later tracheal stenosis. Tracheostomy may be required in obstructive sleep apnoea to bypass the site of air flow obstruction in the pharynx but nocturnal nasal positive airway pressure is an effective alternative

8. Diaphragmatic pacing is rarely used but can be effective particularly after high cervical cord injuries.

Abnormal patterns of respiration

The wide variety of normal patterns of respiration is determined by both reflex factors such as chemoreceptor drive and by behavioural factors such as emotion, exertion etc. However there are some specific respiratory patterns which usually denote disease of the central nervous system.

— *Cheyne-Stokes respiration* is a cyclical waxing and waning of the tidal volume while the respiratory rate remains constant. There may or may not be an apnoeic pause between cycles of Cheyne-Stokes respiration. This type of breathing may occur in normal people during sleep, or in infancy and old age, but is usually associated with a slow circulation time as a result of low cardiac output, or with brain stem ischaemia

— *Central neurogenic hyperventilation* is characterised by rapid respiration (often around 60 per minute) with a fixed large tidal volume. It is due to pontine disease and indicates a poor prognosis

— *Apneustic respiration* is characterised by a deep inspiration followed by prolonged apnoea at a high lung volume and then by slow expiration. It usually indicates medullary disease

— *Gasping respiration* is often a pre-terminal event in patients with severe medullary disease

— *Apnoea.* Quite prolonged periods of apnoea occur, particularly during sleep, when there is either a disorder of the automatic respiratory control system or airflow obstruction in the pharynx or larynx. The profound hypoxia which may develop during these apnoeic periods is often complicated by cardiac dysrhythmias which may be fatal.

29. CHRONIC BRONCHITIS AND EMPHYSEMA

Whilst patients are occasionally seen with apparently pure forms of either chronic bronchitis or emphysema, usually the two conditions coexist to a varying degree in the same patient.

Chronic bronchitis is characterised by chronic production of sputum. A widely used definition requires that cough and sputum occurs on most days for 3 months of the year for at least 3 years. Airflow obstruction is not necessarily present and many, perhaps the majority, of patients in the community with chronic bronchitis have cough and sputum without breathlessness.

Emphysema is characterised pathologically by destruction of alveolar walls with enlargement of air spaces in the lung. Even quite severe emphysema may not be apparent clinically or on X-ray. Symptoms arise as a result of airflow obstruction.

Causes

— Cigarette smoking is the single most important factor in the development of both chronic bronchitis and emphysema

— Atmospheric pollution contributes to the higher prevalence of chronic bronchitis and emphysema in urban compared with rural environments

— Some occupations such as steel manufacture and slate or coal mining are associated with an increased prevalence of chronic bronchitis and emphysema

— Genetic predisposition in the form of deficiency of alpha 1 antitrypsin leads to an increased risk of emphysema which is further increased by smoking

— Some non-pulmonary conditions such as ulcerative colitis can occasionally be associated with chronic cough and purulent sputum even in non-smokers but the nature of this 'bronchitis-like' condition is unknown.

DIAGNOSIS

Symptoms

— *Chronic cough*, usually an early morning 'smokers cough',
and mucoid sputum may be the only symptoms of chronic
bronchitis

— *Increasing breathlessness* on exertion reflects developing
airflow obstruction. It usually comes on gradually and
worsens slowly over several years

— *Recurrent acute bronchitis*, usually in the winter.

The diagnosis of chronic bronchitis or emphysema should be considered
only in present or previous cigarette smokers. It is unwise and unsafe to
diagnose these conditions in non-smokers, light smokers or in young
people who have smoked cigarettes for only a few years.

Signs

Chronic bronchitis and emphysema without airflow obstruction may cause
no abnormal physical signs. When airflow obstruction develops the signs
are similar in chronic bronchitis and in emphysema (see Chapter 5).

Investigations

— *The chest X-ray* may be normal. Severe emphysema causes
an increase in lung volume, reduction of vascular markings, a
narrow heart shadow and sometimes bullae but bullae may
occur in lungs with little general emphysema. The appearance
of the lungs may remain normal in chronic bronchitis even
when severe airflow obstruction has developed but as
pulmonary hypertension develops the proximal portions of the
pulmonary arteries enlarge

— *Lung function tests* may show evidence of airflow obstruction
and where emphysema is predominant the gas transfer for
carbon monoxide is reduced (see Chapter 7). Some
improvement of airflow obstruction is often obtained after
bronchodilator therapy but this is usually less than is typical of
asthma

— *Alpha-1-antitrypsin levels* in serum should be measured in
patients whose emphysema becomes apparent before the age
of 50, who have siblings with the disease or who have
predominantly lower zone changes on chest X-ray. A level
below 20% of normal suggests that the patient is a
homozygote for the deficiency, but Pi typing is then required
for confirmation. Levels greater than 20% are probably of no
relevance to development of emphysema.

Differential diagnosis

— *Asthma* Increasing breathlessness in a cigarette smoker may be due to asthma rather than, or in addition to, chronic bronchitis or emphysema. Because of the possibilities for effective treatment the importance of recognising asthma cannot be over-emphasised. An approach to reaching this diagnosis is discussed in Chapter 30.
— *Bronchiectasis* (see Chapter 22) may cause chronic cough and sputum and, if extensive, breathlessness with airflow obstruction.

TREATMENT

No treatment can restore the destroyed alveoli of emphysema or the damaged airways of chronic bronchitis. Treatment is directed to relief of symptoms and to prevent worsening of the disease.

1. Stopping smoking. Cough and sputum rapidly diminish when the patient stops smoking. The rapid decline in FEV_1 with age seen in smokers can be slowed by stopping smoking. Consistent and repeated medical advice persuades some patients with chronic bronchitis and emphysema to give up smoking. Other aids such as nicotine containing chewing gum are at present under trial. Whatever method or methods are used, repeated attempts should be made to persuade these patients to stop smoking

2. Bronchodilator therapy along the lines recommended for treatment of asthma (see Chapter 30) usually improves breathlessness to some extent even in the absence of any increase of FEV_1 or peak flow. It has been suggested that atropine-like agents such as ipratropium bromide may be particularly effective in chronic bronchitis and these can be used alone or together with adrenergic bronchodilators or oral theophyllines

3. Over-weight patients may become much less brathless after weight reduction

4. Corticosteroids are usually of no benefit to patients with chronic bronchitis or emphysema but can produce dramatic improvement in some, so much so that the diagnosis would then appear to be chronic asthma rather than (or in addition to) chronic bronchitis. A response to steroids cannot be predicted with certainty from clinical or other features so we believe that any patient who is breathless with apparent chronic bronchitis or emphysema should have a therapeutic trial of oral steroids. This is especially the case if:

a. Breathlessness developed or increased suddenly
b. Sputum is absent or scanty or has not been purulent
c. Attacks of cough and breathlessness occur at night
d. Exacerbations occur in summer
e. FEV_1 or PEFR increase by more than 15% after inhalation of a bronchodilator
f. There is a blood eosinophilia.

The procedure for a trial of steroids is described in Chapter 30 where the importance of repeated measurement of lung function before and during the trial is emphasised.

If a response is obtained treatment is continued along the lines recommended for chronic asthma (see Chapter 30)

5. Mucolytic or expectorant agents are, in our view, of little more than placebo value in most patients
6. Influenza immunisation in the autumn is advisable and may reduce the risk of an exacerbation during influenza outbreaks.

COMPLICATIONS IN PATIENTS WITH CHRONIC BRONCHITIS AND EMPHYSEMA

Acute bronchitis

Acute exacerbation of chronic bronchitis usually occurs in the winter, often following a, presumed viral, upper respiratory infection. Sputum, previously mucoid, may become purulent or the volume of previously purulent sputum may increase. Breathlessness may or may not increase but there is often no fever or other systemic upset. FEV_1 or PEFR may fall. Bilateral expiratory wheeze, often varying with coughing, may be the only abnormal sign. Alternatively patients who were previously breathless may become severely ill with tachypnoea, cyanosis and features of repiratory failure (see Chapter 16).

All patients admitted to hospital in exacerbations should have a chest X-ray to exclude pneumonia, pneumothorax or heart failure (signs of which may be difficult to recognise in a wheezing or breathless patient). Those who are ill should have measurement of arterial blood gases to detect respiratory failure (see below). Microbiological examination of sputum is not helpful unless the sputum remains purulent despite recent appropriate antibiotic therapy.

Treatment
1. Increased inhaled bronchodilator may lessen airflow obstruction. This is conveniently given by nebulization in hospital (see Chapter 30)
2. Antibiotics. Mild attacks may improve without antibiotic treatment, but it is customary to treat episodes in which

sputum is purulent with an antibiotic. *H. influenza* and
Strep. pneumoniae are so consistently grown from sputum
under these circumstances that their presence can be assumed
without seeking laboratory confirmation. Ampicillin,
amoxycillin, tetracycline, erythromycin or cotrimoxazole are
equally effective given by mouth for 7 days. Newer antibiotics
such a cephalosporins seem to offer no advantage and are
often more expensive. Laboratory examination of sputum
may be helpful in patients who have not responded to one
course of antibiotics. In general however gram-negative
organisms found in such sputum are contaminants from the
upper respiratory tract and do not usually require speicific
treatment. However sick the patient may be antibiotics offer
no further benefit when the sputum has become mucoid.

Pneumonia

Pneumonia (see also Chapter 18) is a common complication. Diagnosis
may be difficult as, without a chest X-ray and with few if any of the
classic physical signs of consolidation, the clinical picture may differ little
from a severe exacerbation of chronic bronchitis. In patients who are
often immobile and may be oedematous the alternative possibility of
pulmonary embolism to account for symptoms and X-ray changes must be
kept in mind.

Respiratory failure (see Chapter 16)

Suspect respiratory failure in a patient with:
— cyanosis
— confusion or drowsiness
— early morning headache
— tremulousness.
Diagnosis (and treatment) are based on arterial blood gas analysis (see
Chapters 8 & 16) Any of the four main patterns of respiratory failure
may occur:
— *Acute hypoxia without hypercapnia* suggests pneumonia but
may occur during a severe exacerbation of bronchitis without
evident lung consolidation
— *Chronic hypoxia without hypercapnia* may be present for
months or years and is usually worsened during acute
exacerbations of purulent sputum
— *Acute hypercapnia* may develop during a severe exacerbation
in a patient who previously had normal arterial CO_2 tension
— *Chronic hypercapnea* may have been recognised before an
acute illness or may become apparent only when arterial
blood is analysed during an exacerbation.

The importance for therapy of recognising not only the presence of respiratory failure but also the type and severity is discussed in Chapter 16. Management of respiratory failure is discussed in Chapter 16.

Cor pulmonale

Right ventricular hypertrophy (cor pulmonale) and failure develop in some patients with chronic obstructive bronchitis and emphysema. The more severe the airflow obstruction the more likely it is that right ventricular function will deteriorate. It is increasingly recognised that nocturnal hypoventilation during sleep may result in periods of hypoxia and pulmonary hypertension which contribute to the development of cor pulmonale in such patients (see Chapter 16).

Suspect cor pulmonale in a patient with severe airflow obstruction and hypoxia if there is:
— Ankle oedema (this can however occur in patients with chronic hypoxia and/or hypercapnea who do not have raised venous pressure; the mechanism is not understood)
— Raised jugular venous pressure
— Right ventricular heave and an accentuated pulmonary component of the second heart sound.
— Right bundle branch block, right ventricular hypertrophy or right axis deviation on ECG.

Treatment
1. Inhaled bronchodilators (see Chapter 30)
2. Diuretics (digitalis is probably of little or no value in the absence of atrial fibrillation)
3. Long-term oxygen therapy (see Chapter 39 and below).

THE SEVERELY DISABLED PATIENT ('RESPIRATORY CRIPPLE')

Some patients with severe chronic bronchitis and emphysema become disabled by breathlessness. In both diseases the structural damage to the lungs is by then so severe that no major improvement of lung function is possible.

The following questions should be examined before considering the forms of supportive therapy described below:
— Has every effort been made to identify and treat any reversible element of airflow obstruction? Has the patient had a trial of corticosteroids or of high dose inhaled bronchodilators?
— Has right or left heart failure, if present, been treated?
— Might some of the disability be due to recurrent pulmonary embolism?

— Is there severe secondary polycythaemia (Hb over 20 grams per dl, haematcrit over 60%) in which case should venesection by considered?

— Is depression contributing to the disability?

Oxygen therapy (see also Chapter 40)

Oxygen is commonly prescribed for such patients but may be unhelpful or unsafe and is expensive.

— *Occasional intermittent oxygen* used when a patient is particularly breathless is rarely of more than psychological value

— *Portable oxygen* is available in small cylinders which can be filled from larger cylinders and carry enough oxygen for 1–2 hours at low flow of 2–4 litres per minute (systems using liquid oxygen are under trial). The weight of the cylinder to some extent counters the advantage of inhaling oxygen during exercise but there is no doubt that some patients can achieve more exercise while breathing oxygen. The likely benefit for any patient cannot be predicted except by measuring the distance which can be walked with and without oxygen and we recommend such a formal assessment before this troublesome and expensive form of treatment is prescribed

— *Long-term oxygen therapy* is intended to reverse (or prevent) pulmonary hypertension in patients with severe hypoxia. To be effective not less than 15 hours of oxygen inhalation is necessary in every 24 hours which makes considerable demands on the patient and the family. Studies suggest that this treatment may prolong survival in carefully selected patients. At present nocturnal oxygen therapy should be considered only for patients with severe airflow obstruction, who have arterial hypoxaemia, who have stopped smoking, and who do not develop a rise of arterial CO_2 while receiving oxygen.

Introduction of the oxygen concentrator will reduce the cost and the practical difficulties of long-term domiciliary oxygen therapy but this treatment will remain suitable for only a small proportion of patients with severe disease and careful expert assessment is advisable before embarking on this life long treatment

Physical training

This has been advocated as a means of increasing the exercise capacity of severely breathless patients. Small improvements have been demonstrated but the treatment is demanding on staff and time, and is likely to be suitable for only a small proportion of patients. Breathing exercises in themselves have not been shown to be helpful.

Drug treatment of breathlessness

There has been an as yet unsuccessful search for drugs which will safely treat the sensation of breathlessness in patients whose lung function cannot be improved. Minor improvement has been obtained in some patients with small doses of diazepam or dihydrocodeine, but we do not recommend use of these drugs, which may depress respiration, without expert advice.

IPPB

Intermittent positive pressure breathing through a mouthpiece or mask has not been shown to be of value.

Psychological and social support

Breathlessness is markedly influenced by mood and formal studies have shown that anxiety or depression increase the sensation of breathlessness and reduce exercise capacity. In the patient with severe breathlessness psychological factors may be at least as important as lung function in determining disability. Every effort should be made to relieve or treat these factors.

Social support and help with the practical problems of daily living may contribute more than any form of respiratory therapy. Rehousing to avoid stairs or hills, walking aids and every possible financial aid can lessen the burden of the late stages of this disease.

30. ASTHMA

'Generalised airflow obstruction which varies either spontaneously or in response to treatment'. This can develop at any age from childhood to old age.

The patient with airflow obstruction may describe:
— Wheezing
— Tightness
— Breathlessness
— Cough

Symptoms are usually intermittent and it is this which usually suggests the diagnosis of asthma. However, because of this intermittency, the patient may have no abnormal physical signs when seen by a doctor and at these times tests of lung function may be normal.

On the other hand asthma may be persistent in which case the diagnosis may be overlooked especially if there seems to be another possible cause for breathlessness, such as chronic bronchitis or suspected heart disease.

DIAGNOSIS

Consider the diagnosis of asthma in a patient of any age with:
— Episodic wheeze, 'tightness' or breathlessness
— Persistent wheeze, tightness or breathlessness
— Recurrent or paroxysmal cough.

Satisfactory management can only be based on a certain diagnosis and confirmation of the diagnosis is therefore necessary.

To confirm the diagnosis. Evidence is required of both (a) airflow obstruction and (b) variability (Fig. 30.1).

History alone sufficient for diagnosis

A convincing history of recurrent wheeze (usually but not always causing breathlessness) may be sufficient for a confident diagnosis, especially if any of the common predisposing or precipitating factors listed below are present, such as atopy or symptoms provoked by exercise or upper respiratory infection.

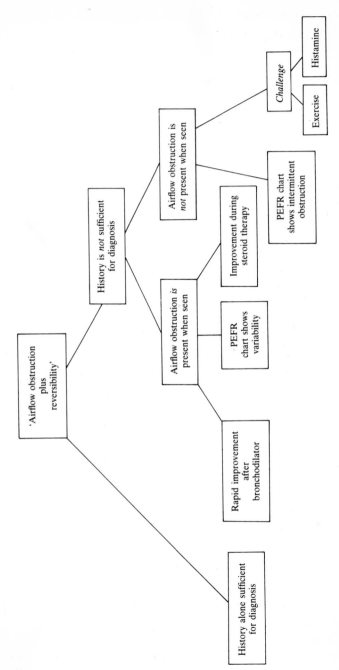

Fig. 30.1

History alone insufficient for diagnosis

In other situations the approach to confirming the diagnosis depends on whether features of airflow obstruction are present when the patient is seen.

Airflow obstruction is present (low FEV_1 or PEFR)

1. Effect of bronchodilator. Increase of FEV_1 or PEFR by more than 20% within 15 minutes of inhaling two puffs of an adrenergic bronchodilator confirms the diagnosis of asthma. If there is less response, or no response, to bronchodilator and if there is no urgency for treatment
2. Measure variability of airflow obstruction:
    a. *Spontaneous*. Serial PEFR records – the patient borrows a peak flow meter and records the best of three peak flow measurements every morning and several times during the day, for at least a week, with extra measurements at times when symptoms are present. A difference of more than 20% between the lowest and the highest PEFR confirms the diagnosis of asthma
    b. *Therapeutic*. If airflow obstruction is present and little variability is detected a therapeutic trial of corticosteroids follows:
        (i) *Oral*. PEFR is recorded, as above, for at least a week after which prednisolone 30 mg daily is given, all other treatment, if any, being continued unchanged. PEFR records are continued. An increase of PEFR greater than 20% is usually apparent within 1 week if the patient has asthma, but improvement may occasionally occur after 2 or 3 weeks if symptoms have been present for a long time previously.

        It is unsafe to judge the response to steroids on changes of symptoms alone unless the response is dramatic and complete, because of the non-specific feeling of well-being and improvement of any symptoms which can occur at the onset of systemic steroid therapy
        (ii) *Inhaled*. If symptoms are not severe a carefully monitored trial of inhaled corticosteroids together with inhaled bronchodilator may be sufficient for diagnosis. After PEFR records for a week regular full dosage of inhaled steroid and bronchiodilators are taken for at least 2 weeks, PEFR being recorded throughout.

No airflow obstruction is present (PEFR or FEV_1 are normal)

Look for episodic airflow obstruction

Serial measurements of PEFR several times a day as above, may show variations of more than 20% either spontaneously (often with a low

PEFR in the early morning) or in response to activities such as exercise or changes in environment. Depending on the pattern of asthma in the individual such falls of PEFR may occur daily or less frequently or perhaps only with upper respiratory infections.

Attempt to provoke airflow obstruction
This can be achieved by exercise or inhalation challenge.

Exercise. The most widely available method of provocation is an exercise test. This is easier to perform on children or young adults than on older adults.

After several 'baseline' measurements of PEFR the patient exercises hard for 6 minutes, either by free running on the flat or on a bicycle ergometer, or laboratory treadmill. PEFR is recorded every 2 minutes after the end of exercise for 20 minutes. A fall of PEFR greater than 20% is characteristic of asthma. Improvement thereafter is usually spontaneous but can be hastened by inhalation of an adrenergic bronchodilator. Unless the test is supervised lack of response may be due to insufficient exertion.

Histamine or methacoline inhalation. This is rarely required for diagnosis and can be carried out safely only in a laboratory by experienced personnel. After several 'baseline' measurements of PEFR or FEV_1 increasing concentrations of histamine or methacholine are inhaled from a nebuliser. Measurements are repeated shortly after each inhalation and the concentration (dose) of agent required to bring about a fall of 20% calculated. Such a fall occurs at a lower concentration in asthmatics than in most non-asthmatics. However some non-asthmatic subjects may respond to a low concentration especially if they are suffering from hay fever or an upper respiratory infection at the time of the test; thus such tests support a diagnosis of asthma but do not prove it.

In practice the diagnosis of asthma is usually made without the need for more demanding tests than measurement of the response to bronchodilator or serial measurements of PEFR. Provocation tests are rarely required.

SOME CAUSES OF ASTHMA

The underlying cause of asthma is not known. It is however helpful to try to answer for each patient:

— What factors contribute to this patient being asthmatic? (predisposing factors)
— What factors precipitate attacks of asthma? ('triggers').

Predisposing factors

Atopy
About 25% of the population of UK is atopic. Such subjects can be

recognised either clinically by symptoms such as seasonal rhinitis (hayfever), or eczema, or immunologically by demonstrating either positive skin prick test reactions to one or more common allergens (see Chapter 14) or raised levels of 1gE in serum. Most childhood or young adult asthmatics are atopic but the majority of those who develop asthma in middle life or later are not atopic.

Family history

A family history of asthma is frequently obtained. It seems that this is not confined to a family history of atopy, for asthma is also disproportionately common in families of non-atopic subjects who have asthma.

'Triggers' of asthma (precipitating factors)

The asthmatic is characterised by increased bronchial reactivity, i.e. a tendency for the airways to be abnormally sensitive to various non-specific stimuli (it is this increased reactivity which is identified in diagnostic tests such as serial measurements of PEFR, exercise tests or histamine challenge).

Whatever the basis for an asthmatic patient's increased bronchial reactivity, bronchoconstriction may be provoked by many quite different stimuli ('triggers'). Hence an atopic subject with predominantly summer asthma related to grass pollens may develop an attack of asthma also after exercise (in the pollen season or outside it), or after a winter upper respiratory infection. Different attacks may be provoked by different 'triggers'.

Some common or important 'triggers' of asthma

Exercise

Asthma, particularly in the young, is often precipitated by exercise and this is the basis for the exercise test used in diagnosis. Symptoms tend to follow a short spell of hard exercise but may occur during the course of more prolonged exercise.

Air temperature

Inhalation of cold, dry air often provokes asthma and some patients may describe wheezing on changing from a cold to a warm atmosphere.

Seasons

Seasons may influence asthma by their effect on air temperature, by the occurrence of upper respiratory infection or by seasonal air-borne allergens (see below).

Allergies

The commonest domestic allergens contributing to asthma are furry pets and house dust, but it may not be easy to recognise or prove the relationship. Dander from animals becomes widely spread in a house and symptoms may continue after temporary removal of the animal. The allergen in house dust derives particularly from the house dust mite

(Dermatophagoides) which is most prolific in autumn and winter. Seasonal allergens include tree pollens (spring), grass pollens (summer), moulds (autumn) and many others.

Occupation
See Chapter 36).

Food and drink
Asthma usually occurs soon after ingestion, and may be due to preservatives (sulphur dioxide in drinks and some packaged foods), colouring agents (especially tartrazine in many foods and drinks) or impurities (e.g. resins and other substances in wines). The role of true 'food allergy' is uncertain, except in a few obvious situations when asthma follows immediately after a particular food.

Emotions
Emotional disturbance may act, like other 'triggers', to precipitate attacks in those who are already asthmatic, but there is no reason to think either that emotional disturbances are an underlying cause of asthma or that asthmatics have more of these disturbances than non-asthmatics.

Drugs
Beta blocking drugs will worsen pre-existing asthma but do not cause it in previously non-asthmatic people. Analgesics (mainly but not solely aspirin) may precipate asthma especially in older patients who also have nasal polypi.

Upper respiratory infections
These are a common trigger of exacerbations of asthma.
   Note: Symptoms may be wrongly attributed to 'chest infection' rather than asthma, but such episodes respond to, and are prevented by, conventional asthma therapy, without any treatment for infection.

INVESTIGATION OF ASTHMA

Chest X-ray

This is usually normal between acute attacks unless the asthma is severe and prolonged (when over-inflation and bronchial wall thickening may develop) or unless complications such as bronchopulmonary aspergillosis have developed (see below).

Blood count

The blood count is usually normal. Eosinophilia (up to 1000 mm^2) is not uncommon in either atopic or non-atopic asthmatics, but may be intermittent. Higher levels raise the possibility of pulmonary eosinophilia (see later) or vasculitis.

Skin tests

Prick skin tests (see Chapter 14) are not, in our opinion, useful as a routine and are rarely a guide to treatment. They can be used to demonstrate atopy. When the diagnosis of asthma is being considered as a possibility, the presence of atopy will perhaps add weight to the diagnosis. Skin tests may also be used to support and add emphasis to advice on, for example, removal of pets from a household. They are a necessary preliminary to consideration of hyposensitisation.

Differential diagnosis of asthma

Recent wheezing

Other causes of obstruction of the airways should be considered:
- *In a young child* – inhaled foreign body (see Chapter 24)
- *In an older person* – endobronchial or endotracheal tumour (see Chapter 31).

Long-standing wheezy breathlessness
- *In a young person or child* – cystic fibrosis (see Chapter 23)
- *In a smoker* – chronic bronchitis and emphysema (see Chapter 29)
- *With persistent purulent sputum* – widespread bronchiectasis (see Chapter 22).

GENERAL PRINCIPLES IN THE MANAGEMENT OF ASTHMA

Is there an avoidable cause?

Before embarking on drug therapy, which can only relieve or suppress asthma, consider the possibility of an avoidable cause. Many factors such as pollens, animals, house dust, foods, drinks, drugs, upper respiratory infections etc, act as triggers for asthma in those with hyper-reactive airways but are not in themselves the cause of the asthmatic state. Avoidance, when possible, may improve but is unlikely to abolish the asthma.

If there is good evidence, from a carefully taken history, of such triggers then attempts to reduce exposure are worth trying. Vaccum cleaning and using a damp duster may reduce inhalation of house dust as may covering a mattress with a plastic sheet and removing excessive soft furnishings from bedrooms. Furry pets and birds should usually be banished from the house of an atopic asthmatic unless the asthma is controlled by simple treatment or great distress would be caused by the loss of the pets.

In practice, cure of asthma is virtually confined to removal of occupational causes hence their great importance (see Chapter 36).

Drug therapy

Drug therapy is needed for most patients with asthma. The available drugs fall into several categories:

Bronchodilators

Adrenergic
Earlier agents such as adrenaline, isoprenaline or ephedrine are no longer used having been superceded by the more selective beta 2 adrenergic agents. Many agents are now available of which the most widely used are salbutamol, terbutaline, fenoterol and rimiterol.
   These are generally best given by inhalation because:
   — The dose required is smaller than by mouth and side effects are fewer
   — The onset of action is faster than by mouth
   — The duration of action is as long as by mouth.
Most can also be given by I.V. or I.M. injection. Muscle tremor or palpitations may occur at high dosage or in unusually susceptible subjects.
   Safety. There is a very wide margin of safety for these drugs inhaled from aerosols or other hand-held devices. Warnings about exceeding the recommended dose are unfounded and patients should be encouraged to use the quantity required to relieve symptoms. If large doses are needed this shows the need for other forms of treatment (see below).

Atropine-like
Atropine itself is rarely used but ipratropium bromide is available from a pressurised aerosol. Side effects are few at usual dosage.

Theophyllines
These act by a different mechanism from adrenergic or atropine-like bronchodilators. Oral theophyllines have long suffered from problems of a narrow therapeutic range and the risk of intolerance or toxicity. Long acting and slow release preparations have gone some way to overcoming these problems. Many preparations are available, each with different dosage schedules. Aminophylline may be given by intravenous injection. At excessive dosage tremor, confusion, nausea, vomiting, cardiac arrthymias or sudden death may occur.

Prophylactic agents
   — *Disodium cromoglycate* (DSCG – Intal) acts only as a prophylactic and has no bronchodilator activity. Hence it must be taken regularly or before exposure to provoking factors such as exercise. It is taken only by inhalation. There are no important side effects. Powder, aerosol or nebulised preparations are available
   — *Inhaled corticosteroids* have prophylactic action in asthma. At the usual dose absorption is trivial and there are no systemic side effects. Oral candidiasis may occurs but is usually readily controlled with nystatin. The voice may become hoarse. There is no increased risk of pulmonary infection. At high

doses such as 2000 µg of beclomethaone, slight adrenal-pituitary suppression can be demonstrated
— *Systemic corticosteroids* are given by mouth, usually as prednisolone, or intravenously as hydrocortisone. The risk of adverse effects of prolonged high dosage are well known but are reduced by alternative day therapy.

Other drugs

Antihistamines
Taken by mouth, these are of no value in treatment of asthma, in spite of their good effect in allergic rhinitis.

Antibiotics
These are of no value unless there is evidence of bacterial or mycoplasma infection, which is rarely the case.

Sedatives or anti-anxiety drugs
These have no beneficial effects and may be dangerous in severe asthma.

Ketotifen
This seems to be of little value.

'Vaccines'
Attempts to 'desensitise' against one or more allergens have been disappointing when subjected to rigorous clinical trial. They involve repeated courses of injections and carry a risk of anaphylaxis. However improvement has been claimed in patients whose asthma is provoked only, or mainly, by a single recognisable allergen. Even when this seems to be the case our preference is generally for drug therapy and experience with vaccines against grass pollens or house dust mite have generally been disappointing in the treatment of asthma (although more effective in treating rhinitis).

Use of inhalers and inhaler devices

Many forms of asthma therapy are best delivered by inhalation, but not all patients can or will use inhalers to their best effect. *It cannot be assumed that an inhaler once prescribed will be used correctly, and explanation and demonstration are necessary for patients of any age and of any level of intelligence.*

How to use a pressurised aerosol
1. Remove the cover and shake the inhaler
2. Holding the inhaler vertically with the mouth piece lowermost, breathe out gently and then
3. Place the mouth piece in the mouth, and close the lips around it. After starting to breathe in slowly and deeply through the mouth, press the inhaler firmly to release the aerosol
4. Hold the breath while counting to 10, then breathe out slowly.

If more than one puff is required repeat the sequence as above. Aerosols containing placebo are available for tuition and explanation and most, but not all, patients can learn to use pressurised aerosols adequately. Problems remain for some, especially young children and the elderly or disabled. For these, other devices have been produced.

'Spacers'
The insertion of a reservoir between the pressurised aerosol mouth piece and the patient's mouth not only reduces the need to coordinate inhalation with pressing the inhaler but seems to increase the dose of aerosol reaching the lungs and hence to increase effectiveness. Small spacers as an extension of the aerosol device or larger pear-shaped reservoirs are now available for some preparations.

Dry powder inhalers
The agent is mixed with an inert powder in a capsule which is severed or punctured in a special device and then inhaled from the mouth piece. No special coordination is required.

Nebulisers (see also Chapter 40)
These allow larger doses of drug to be delivered with even less need for coordination by the patient. Their main application in the treatment of asthma at present is in delivery bronchodilator agents in treatment of severe asthma, and of prophylactic agents in treating very young children.

Combined drug inhalers
The frequent need for patients to use more than one type of inhaler has led to various combinations in a single inhaler. We do not recommend use of combined cromoglycate with isoprenaline as this frequently leads to inappropriate use for its bronchodilator action alone. Likewise we are not impressed with the benefits of combining inhaled steroids with bronchodilators. The combination of two different types of bronchodilator, fenoterol and ipratropium, may have some practical advantages. The use of fixed combinations discourages the prescriber form varying the dosage of each agent, which is often the best approach to therapy.

PRACTICAL MANAGEMENT OF THE ASTHMATIC PATIENT

Occasional asthma

This is best relieved by inhalation of an adrenergic bronchodilator such as salbutamol, terbutalene etc. Two puffs (with separate inhalations) is the usual dose for an adult or older child, one puff for a younger child, but larger doses than this carry no risk of toxicity, unless used repeatedly because of a poor response (see below). The same treatment before exertion can be used to prevent exercise induced asthma.

Frequent or continuous asthma

Inhaled adrenergic bronchodilators, as above, can be taken regularly 4–6 times daily but it is usually more satisfactory to the patient to take regular prophylaxis in an attempt to prevent symptoms. The choice of prophylaxis rests between cromoglycate which is usually the initial choice for children, or inhaled corticosteroids.

Cromoglycate must be taken 4 times a day whereas corticosteroids are effective taken only twice a day, a considerable practical advantage. There is no advantage in combining cromoglycate and inhaled steroids and, in general, inhaled steroids are the more effective.

It is essential that the patient understands that these prophylactic agents are intended to prevent and not to relieve asthma and that they must be taken regularly. Most such patients also need inhaled bronchodilators at times, often on walking, but we do not, in general, favour the use of combined preparations (see above).

Oral theophyllines are of special value for preventing nocturnal or early morning asthma. Long-acting preparations taken at night may be effective but it is difficult to establish the right dose. Some recommend 'tailoring' the dose to each individual by measuring blood levels of theophylline at different dosage and this may be the only way of avoiding under dosage which is ineffective or, more important, overdosage which is potentially dangerous.

Worsening of asthma should be treated first by extra doses of inhaled bronchodilator. Several extra doses can be taken with safety. *Patients should be warned not to take extra doses of oral theophyllines.* If additional doses of bronchodilator are not effective and if asthma persists the patient needs a short course of oral prednisolone. Increasing the dose of an inhaled steroid is usually ineffective and may be harmful by delaying the start of oral therapy. For an adult 30 mg prednisolone on the first day is usually adequate and the dose can usually be reduced by 5 mg each day thereafter. Antibiotics are of no value in this situation.

Most patients with more than slight asthma who require regular therapy should have a small supply of prednisolone tablets for 'emergency' use. Such patients should be told, and reminded from time to time:

      — under which circumstances oral prednisolone should be taken
      — the starting dose and the dose thereafter
      — how to gauge the response
      — how to recognise a severe attack (see p 168).

With this information most asthmatics should be able to make their own decision about courses of oral steroids, hence avoiding the delays of seeking medical advice at the time of an attack. Patients who have frequent attacks may be helped in this decision by regular peak flow measurements.

Persistent troublesome asthma while taking regular therapy

1. Peak flow records over several weeks are valuable to show the severity and the pattern of the asthma
2. Confirm that therapy is being taken as recommended and that the technique of using inhalers is adequate
3. If symptoms are severe, or peak flow low, a short course of oral predinisolone may bring about improvement. Prednisolone 30 mg daily for a week is usually sufficient. After such a course, improvement can often be maintained by the same inhaled steroid and bronchodilator therapy that was previously ineffective. Alternatively a higher dose of inhaled corticosteroid can be given. An aerosol containing 250 μg/puff of beclomethasone compared with 50 μg/puff of the conventional aerosol is now available. Up to 8 puffs daily (4 puffs b.d.) may be very effective but at this dose there is some evidence of absorption and slight adreno-pituitary suppression
4. Some patients require regular oral steroid therapy despite other measures. The dose required should be established by daily records of PEFR. Such patients should also take high doses of inhaled corticosteroids to minimise the dosage of prednisolone.

    If long term oral steroids are required side effects are reduced by taking an equivalent dose on alternate days (e.g. 30 mg on alternate days instead of 15 mg daily). An occasional patient may find alternate day therapy less effective in which case a small dose may be given one day and a larger one on the next.
5. Some patients with persisting severe asthma or with occasional sudden severe attacks may benefit from a nebuliser at home from which they can inhale large doses of bronchodilator. Because of the practical difficulties of providing, maintaining and sterilising nebulisers in the home, their cost and the anxieties about the safety of very high doses of bronchodilators (used without supervision), we believe that home nebuliser bronchodilator therapy should be offered only to patients who have failed to respond to other forms of treatment.

Severe acute asthma

In spite of over 1000 deaths annually from asthma in the UK, many in young people, clinicians have been slow to accept that attacks of asthma may be fatal. Most deaths in the home or in hospital are still due to inadequate treatment, usually because the severity of the attack, and hence the risk, has not been appreciated by the patient or, all too often, by the doctor.

How severe is this attack?

Great harm was done by the term 'status asthmaticus' which for many years was used synonymously with 'dangerous asthma' and was defined as an attack which persists for 24 hours. In fact about three quarters of all asthma deaths occur within 24 hours of the onset of the final attack, and about 20% within 2 hours. The duration of an attack is but one measure of its severity and by no means the most important.

Signs of severe asthma

History

> — Inability to speak fluently*
> — Confusion*
> — Inability to sleep because of asthma*
> — Lack of response to inhaled bronchodilator drugs which were previously effective*

Examination

> — Cyanosis*
> — Rapid pulse*
> — Pulsus paradoxus (over 10 mmHg) difference is systolic blood pressure between inspiration and expiration)

Tests

> — PEFR very low*

Any combination of these signs or symptoms indicates a medical emergency which is difficult or impossible to treat safely in the home and usually requires transfer immediately to hospital.

Note: Never delay or refuse immediately hospital admission or consultation for an attack of asthma when this is requested by a patient, a relative, a friend or a doctor.

Note that the features marked above with an asterisk * can easily be noted by the patient or by a non-medical observer and their importance as signs of serious attacks should be understood by all concerned.

Further investigations

Chest X-ray

If the patients' condition allows a chest X-ray (PA only) is advisable to exclude pneumothorax, lobar collapse or pneumomediastinum all of which may be almost impossible to detect clinically during severe asthma.

Arterial blood gases (see Chapter 8)

Hypoxia is invariable in a severe attack. Pa_{CO_2} falls in an asthma attack but, as severity increases, begins to rise. With continued deterioration Pa_{CO_2} reaches a normal level after which it rises further. Hence a raised Pa_{CO_2} (or even a normal Pa_{CO_2}) in a patient with severe asthma is a sign of great severity requiring emergency treatment.

Electrocardiogram

This may abnormal but adds little to assessment in an emergency.

Treatment

1. Patients with severe asthma must be treated in a place where careful and repeated observation by trained staff is possible. Deterioration (and death), may be very sudden and can be anticipated only by close observation

2. *No sedative, hypnotic or analgesic drugs may be given to a patient with severe asthma or fatal respiratory failure may occur*

3. Give oxygen immediately. Abolition of hypoxia is unlikely to cause hypercapnia (except, it is said, in young children) but we recommend a 28% or 35% venturi mask which usually provides sufficient oxygen to achieve a safe Pa_{O_2}

4. Start treatment immediately with a nebulised β2 adrenergic bronchodilator such as salbutamol 5 mg in 4 ml repeated 4-hourly. We prefer inhaled to intravenous bronchodilators

5. Corticosteroids. Give 200–300 mg of hydrocortisone hemisuccinate intravenously immediately because no effect can be expected for several hours. The patient should have received this at home if he saw a doctor before transfer to hospital. This is repeated to give a total dose of at lease 1200 mg in the first 24 hours. Continuous infusion is usually preferred. Prednisolone 30–60 mg daily is started by mouth as soon as possible

6. Correct dehydration. Set up an intravenous infusion to provide fluid and as a route for hydrocortisone. Patients with severe asthma are often dehydrated and may be hypovolaemic, and my be unable to drink freely when very breathless

7. Intravenous aminophylline is an effective broncho-dilator but it is not known whether it produces significant further improvement in addition to high doses of β2 adrenergic agents. If given, the recommended dosage is an initial bolus of 5–6 mg/kg body-weight followed by an I.V infusion of 0.5 mg/kg body-weight per hour or alternatively, and safer, no bolus but an infusion of 0.9 mg/kg per hour. Note that the standard 250 mg ampoule of aminophylline is insufficient for the initial dose in most cases and two ampoules may be excessive. Calculate the dose required.

   Beware! Has the patient recently received oral theophyllines or intravenous aminophylline? The dangers of overdosage are such that aminophylline should be avoided or given with caution if these agents have been used recently. If the patient was given an I.V injection before arriving at hospital or on arrival, was this aminophylline? Many oral asthma treatments contain theophyllines. Patients often take additional tablets during a bad attack, and may not know what they contain. Long-acting tablets may produce blood levels for up to 24 hours. If in doubt it is wise to avoid further aminophylline unless theophylline blood levels can be measured.

8. Assess the response to treatment by frequent measurement of:
   a. Pulse rate (will fall with improvement)
   b. Respiratory rate (will fall with improvement)
   c. Peak flow (will rise)
   d. Arterial blood gases.
   Even when the patient improves, wide diurnal fluctuations of airflow obstruction (PEFR) may persist for several days and during this time the patient may continue to be at risk of sudden death. Corticosteriods and full doses of bronchodilators should be continued during this period and peak flow should be recorded several times a day until stable. Infusion of aminophylline at night may prevent or reduce night time deterioration

9. Assisted ventilation is rarely needed and when it is, this often reflects delayed, inadequate or inappropriate earlier treatment. The surest indication of the need for assisted ventilation is a rising $Paco_2$ but some patients may maintain a 'normal' $Paco_2$ only at the expense of distressing and exhausting ventilatory effort and may need assisted ventilation.

   When a decision is made to ventilate for severe asthma speed is essential (patients have died while awaiting ventilation) and an expert anaesthetist is needed for intubation, which may be very difficult in these circumstances

   During ventilation very high inflation pressures may be needed and there is a risk of pneumothorax or surgical emphysema. When improvement occurs however it is usually rapid and ventilation can often be stopped and the endotracheal tube removed within 24–48 hours. Hence heavy sedation or long-acting muscle paralysis should be avoided if possible

10. What went wrong? Later review is an important and often neglected aspect of treatment of a severe attack of asthma:
    a. Can any avoidable factors be identified, such as failure to take regular therapy, or ingestion of analgesics, beta blockers or certain foods and drinks?
    b. Was treatment modified soon enough and appropriately? Did the patient have a supply of prednisolone to take at the onset of a severe attack?
    c. Was help summoned early enough and, if summoned, was the response adequate?
    This is an ideal time to discuss prevention and management of any future severe attacks with the patient and, if appropriate, with relatives, friends or school teachers.

SOME SPECIAL PROBLEMS

Occupational asthma (see also Chapter 36)

Occupational causes of asthma are of great importance because affected patients may be cured of their asthma but if the cause is not recognised then they may become severely disabled or at least suffer the inconvenience or risks of therapy. All adult patients with asthma should be questioned closely about their work.

Suspect an occupational factor in a patient with asthma if:

— Work involves exposure to a known cause of asthma (see Chapter 36)
— The onset was soon after starting a new job or after a change of process or materials in an old job
— Others at work have developed respiratory symptoms (often wrongly ascribed to 'bronchitis')
— Symptoms improve at weekends or during holidays.

Beware: Occupational asthma, though episodic at the onset, may become persistent with time and patients are often wrongly diagnosed as having chronic bronchitis, especially if they smoke cigarettes. An association with work is then unlikely to be considered and further deterioration may occur. For the investigation and management of occupational asthma see Chapter 36.

Pulmonary eosinophilia (see Chapter 37)

Allergic bronchopulmonary aspergillosis

Allergic bronchopulmonary aspergillosis is the commonest cause in the UK of 'pulmonary eosinophilia' (pulmonary opacities on chest X-ray associated with blood eosinophilia). It is the result of a hypersensitivity reaction to the fungus aspergillus fumigatus which reaches the lungs as inhaled spores. Other causes of pulmonary eosinophilia are discussed in Chapter 37.

Consider allergic bronchopulmonary aspergillosis in a patient with asthma who has:

— Exacerbations particularly in autumn or winter with mucopurulent sputum, or fever or pleuritic pain
— Hard lumps ('plugs') in sputum (which on inspection can be sometimes seen to be casts of bronchi)
— An abnormal chest X-ray. Various appearances may be seen:
  a. Patchy pulmonary opacities, usually of segmental distribution, often multiple and transient or fluctuating
  b. Lobar or segmental collapse
  c. Tubular or ring shadows suggesting bronchiectasis
  d. Loss of volume of upper lobes in long-standing disease.
— Blood eosinophilia.

The diagnosis is supported by:

- — Positive immediate prick skin test to antigen of aspergillus fumigatus occurs in all patients with allergic bronchopulmonary aspergillosis but also in about 15% of atopic subjects without it
- — Precipitins against aspergillus fumigatus are present in the serum of about 70% of patients with allergic aspergillosis, the proportion increasing to 90% if the serum is concentrated
- — A dual (immediate weal followed after some hours by an indurated non-itchy Arthus-type reaction) to intradermal injection of antigen of aspergillus fumigatus. This test is rarely carried out in practice
- — Demonstration of characteristic proximal dilatation of bronchi in previously involved areas of lung on bronchography
- — Raised total IgE levels in serum (useful if the results of other tests have been inconclusive).

In the late stages of the disease, as, for example, when upper lobe fibrosis has developed, precipitins may no longer be present in the serum. Diagnosis is then based on probability and exclusion of other causes of such an appearance.

Management

There is no known way of eliminating aspergillus from the respiratory tract or preventing its entry or colonisation. Oral corticosteroids (prednisolone 30–40 mg daily) are the only means of treating episodes of pulmonary eosinophilia, and the radiological response is usually rapid.

The asthma of patients with allergic bronchopulmonary aspergillosis may often be controlled with conventional inhaled therapy, but the evidence suggests that inhaled steroids to not prevent further episodes of pulmonary eosinophilia although they may mask symptoms. This raises the fear that patients so treated may developed permanent lung damage without warning symptoms.

Continued oral prednisolone in a dose of about 10 mg daily may reduce the frequency of episodes but it is often difficult to advise such indefinite treatment for a patient who may have had only one or two episodes of pulmonary eosinophilia without, as yet, any evidence of permanent damage. Oral steroids do not introduce a risk of disseminated or invasive aspergillus infection in this context.

31. LUNG TUMOURS

Most primary pulmonary tumours are bronchial carcinomas. Other benign or malignant tumours are briefly discussed later in this chapter.

BRONCHIAL CARCINOMA

Bronchial carcinoma should be suspected in a patient over 35 who is or was a cigarette smoker with:

> — *Haemoptysis*. Lung cancer usually causes recurrent streaking or spotting of sputum with blood rather than large haemoptysis
> — *Cough*. This is common in smokers due to chronic bronchitis but with the development of lung cancer the cough may change in character or frequency
> — *Chest pain*. This may be due to involvement of (a) the pleura or the chest wall (giving pleuritic pain or a continuous dull pain), (b) mediastinal lymph nodes (occasionally giving central chest pain), or (c) the brachial plexus giving pain and sensory loss down the inside of the arm (Pancoast syndrome)
> — *Breathlessness*. This may be due to the size of the tumour itself, to pulmonary collapse from bronchial obstruction, to a pleural effusion or to lymphangitis carcinomatosa
> — *Wheeze or stridor*. Obstruction to the trachea or main bronchi may cause stridor. Wheeze due to partial obstruction of a bronchus is usually best heard over the region ventilated through that bronchus
> — *Hoarseness*. This is due to involvement of the left recurrent laryngeal nerve
> — *Recurrent pneumonia* or a single episode which has been slow to clear as a result of bronchial obstruction
> — *Dysphagia*. This may be due to spread of the tumour to the mediastinal lymph nodes or to the oesophagus
> — *Superior vena caval obstruction*

— *Systemic symptoms* such as weight loss, weakness or anorexia which are early symptoms in about 50% of patients with lung cancer

— *Symptoms from metastases*, most frequently in the brain, liver, bones or adrenal glands

— *Non-metastatic effects* such as peripheral neuropathy, dermatomyositis or syndromes mimicking secretion of hormones e.g. ADH, ACTH, PTH.

High risk groups

Suspicion is increased in high risk groups.

— Is the patient a smoker? The risk of developing a bronchial carcinoma (relative to a non-smoker) is increased approximately by the number of cigarettes smoked per day (20 cigarettes per day increases the chance of developing bronchial carcinoma by 20 times)

— Has the patient been exposed to any occupational hazards? Blue asbestos is the most dangerous type of asbestos and was encountered in high concentrations while lagging pipes and boilers and by workers on an asbestos production line. Remember that most carcinogens have a latent period of at least 15 years before the tumour is apparent

— Has the patient diffuse chronic pulmonary fibrosis (cryptogenic fibrosing alveolitis, systemic sclerosis etc)? The risk of lung cancer is increased in these conditions.

Physical signs

The following physical signs increase the suspicion of bronchial carcinoma:

— *Clubbing of the fingers*, with or without hypertrophic osteoarthropathy. The latter is suspected from pain and swelling of the limbs around large joints and can be confirmed by seeing periosteal changes on X-ray

— *Palpable lymph nodes*, particularly in the supraclavicular region. Isolated axillary lymph node enlargement is rarely due to lung cancer.

— *Signs of collapse*, consolidation or pleural effusion may be due to lung cancer but are not specific

— *Stridor* occurs if the trachea or main bronchi are compressed or partially occluded. A unilateral wheeze strongly suggests unilateral bronchial obstruction, commonly by a carcinoma

— *Hoarseness*

— *Superior vena caval obstruction*

— *Sensory loss in arm*, weakness of hypothenar muscles, Horner's syndrome

— *Enlarged and irregular liver*.

— *Signs of metastases* in the brain, bones, skin or elsewhere, which in high risk patients are commonly from a bronchial carcinoma.

Investigations to confirm the diagnosis

Chest X-ray

A chest X-ray may show the tumour itself as a pulmonary mass or cavity. Alternatively it may show changes secondary to bronchial obstruction such as unresolving pneumonia or collapse of a lobe or lung. Secondary changes may include pleural effusion, enlarged hilar or mediastinal lymph nodes. Peripheral tumours may destroy adjacent ribs. An elevated diaphragm suggests tumour involvement of the phrenic nerve. Enlargement of the heart shadow may indicate malignant pericardial effusion.

Note that:
— a normal chest X-ray does not exclude a bronchial carcinoma
— an all-too-common error is to overlook a tumour because no lateral view was obtained
— most peripheral tumours are not visible on the chest X-ray until they are larger than 1 cm diameter. Central tumours may become much larger before they are seen either because they are within the large airways or are 'hidden' in the mediastinum. If a tumour is suspected in the large airways tomograms or oblique views of the trachea may be useful, but bronchoscopy is a more certain method of diagnosis.

Sputum cytology

Cytological examination of sputum confirms the diagnosis in up to 70% of cases but absence of malignant cells does not exclude a carcinoma. An inexperienced cytologist may report false positive results in patients with chronic bronchial inflammation. Remember that malignant cells may arise from the upper airway e.g. from carcinoma of the larynx. Sputum samples for cytology should be received by the laboratory within 2 hours of expectoration. Early morning samples are not required.

Bronchoscopy

Bronchoscopy enables the tumour to be seen in about 70% of cases (see Chapter 10) and biopsy can be obtained to ascertain the cell type. Involvement of the trachea or main carina or compression of the trachea by lymph nodes imply that the tumour is inoperable. Contrary to previous teaching bronchoscopy carries no extra risk in patients with superior vena caval obstruction.

Pleural aspiration and biopsy

These should always be performed if a patient with possible or definite bronchial carcinoma has a pleural effusion. Effusions are not always due to spread of tumour to the pleura but may develop as a reaction to pneumonia beyond a tumour or to lymphatic obstruction. Blood straining of the fluid or rapid reaccummulation after aspiration strongly suggest malignant involvement of the pleura. Cytological examination of pleural fluid is more open to error than cytological examination of sputum.

Percutaneous needle biopsy (see Chapter 11)
This is valuable for diagnosis of peripheral tumours which are difficult to biopsy by the transbronchial technique. In our experience, diagnosis is reached in over 90% of such cases.

Biopsy of suspected metastases
Peripheral lymph nodes can be aspirated with a fine needle and the material examined cytologically. Subcutaneous nodules are readily biopsied with local anaesthesia.

Mediastinoscopy and/or mediastinotomy
Mediastinoscopy or mediastinotomy may be necessary to biopsy enlarged mediastinal lymph nodes if no pulmonary tumour is visible or accessible. They are safe and effective methods of diagnosing the cause of superior vena caval obstruction.

Management

The management of a patient with bronchial carcinoma rests on the following factors:

Cell type
What is the cell type? Small ('oat') cell carcinomas are rarely cured by resection of the primary tumour because micro metastases are nearly always present at the time of diagnosis. Surgical removal may however be considered in the rare event of a peripheral small cell carcinoma being detected without evidence of distant spread.

Surgical resection
If the tumour is not a small cell carcinoma, is surgical resection possible and advisable? Almost all the long-term survivors from lung cancer have had complete removal of their tumour. It is therefore essential to consider both whether resection is likely to be curative and whether lung tissue can be removed without causing severe residual breathlessness. Only one in eight of all patients with lung cancer is found to be operable and of these about one third survive more than 5 years.

Resection is indicated if all four of the following requirements are met:
1. The patient is not too old (usually under 65 for pneumonectomy, under 70 for lobectomy) and is fit enough to withstand a thoracotomy. Other illnesses such as diabetes, coronary artery disease etc, must be taken into account
2. There are no distant metastases. A careful history and examination are essential to detect metastases, and special care should be taken to feel for supraclavicular lymph node enlargement and for hepatomegaly. Routine investigations should include full blood count, liver function tests, blood calcium, phosphate, urea and electrolytes. If any of these are

abnormal of if symptoms or signs suggest metastases, further investigation will be required e.g. bone scan, bone marrow examination, isotope or ultrasound examination of the liver, brain scan or computed tomography. The yield from bone, liver or brain scans is very small in the absence of clinical or biochemical abnormalities, and these should not therefore be considered routine investigations.

3. The tumour is locally operable. Invasion of the mediastinum causing paralysis of the phrenic or recurrent laryngeal nerves, or obstruction of the superior vena cava or oesophageal compression are contraindications to surgery. Pleural effusion effusion usually, but not always, indicates spread to the pleura and hence inoperability. Pleural aspiration and biopsy or occasionally thoracoscopy are advisable before a decision is reached. Direct local invasion of the ribs does not necessarily preclude resection of a tumour, since they can sometimes be resected with the lung tumour.

   Assessment of local operability is based on:
   a. Chest X-ray. Look for mediastinal lymph node enlargement, diaphragmatic paralysis or lymphangitis, all of which indicate inoperability
   b. Findings at bronchoscopy. Widened main carina, tracheal involvement or compression, or vocal cord paralysis indicate inoperability. The need for a lobectomy or pneumonectomy can often be assessed from the site of the tumour
   c. Pleural biopsy and aspiration if an effusion is present
   d. Assessment of mediastinal lymph nodes. Some units perform mediastinoscopy on all patients before reaching a decision on thoracotomy. However computed tomography, if available, will show the presence, size and site of mediastinal lymph nodes. If nodes are less than 1.0 cm in diameter they are unlikely to be malignant and if they are greater than 2.5 cm diameter they almost certainly are malignant. We advise mediastinoscopy or anterior mediastinotomy to biopsy mediastinal nodes of between 1.0 and 2.5 cm diameter. Tumour involvement of mediastinal nodes usually precludes curative surgery.

4. Respiratory function is adequate. It is of course the residual lung function after resection of one or more lobes or of a lung which matters, whereas pre-operative lung function tests examine the function of two lungs. In general, severe breathlessness is unlikely to be a problem after surgery if before operation the patient can climb stairs without stopping and has an FEV_1 greater than 1.5 litres for a pneumonectommy and 1.0 litres for a lobectomy. In border-

line cases a ventilation and perfusion lung scan may show the relative contribution of each lung or an exercise test may clarify how disabled the patient is.

Further treatment

If the patient is not suitable for curative surgery, is further treatment needed? In general patients with non small cell carcinomas who have few or no symptoms rarely benefit in the short-term from radiotherapy or chemotherapy but it is not known whether later distressing symptoms might be prevented or delayed by earlier treatment. Symptoms, when present, can usually be controlled for a time by radiotherapy, chemotherapy, symptomatic drug treatment and occasionally by surgery (Table 31.1).

The median survival of patients with small cell carcinoma without treatment is 3 months from diagnosis but with chemotherapy this can be extended to 18 months in selected cases. Chemotherapy is of no proven benefit in the treatment of squamous and adenocarcinomas, but in small cell carcinomas it gives the best results in patients with limited disease who are young and are otherwise in good general health. It may occasionally be required for palliation but radiotherapy is also very effective in the short-term. A large variety of cytotoxic drug regimes have been used but the most effective drugs, are etoposide (VP 16), cyclophosphamide,

Table 31.1 Palliative treatment for bronchial carcinoma

Complication	Treatment
Haemoptysis	Radiotherapy
Chest wall pain	Radiotherapy
	Indomethacin/opiates
	Surgical resection of ribs; nerve blocks or spinal tract surgery
Pleural effusion	Complete aspiration, then intrapleural tetracycline 500 mg
Bronchial obstruction if causing problems e.g. distal pneumonia, abscess, dyspnoea	Radiotherapy
Dysphagia	Radiotherapy/celestin tube
Vocal cord palsy	Teflon injection into vocal cord
Pericardial tamponade	Construct pericardial window surgically
SVC obstruction	Radiotherapy, or if small cell carcinoma chemotherapy; corticosteroids initially
Pancoast syndrome	Radiotherapy followed by surgical resection
Cerebral metastases	Dexamethasone (plus chemotherapy if small cell carcinoma)
Bone metastases	Radiotherapy plus internal fixation if needed
Spinal cord compression	Emergency decompression followed by radiotherapy. Catheterise, Bowel care
Addisons disease	Hormonal replacement
Neuromyopathy	No effective treatment
Hypertrophic osteoarthropathy	Indomethacin, corticosteroids; Vagotomy, tumour resection
Inappropiate ADH secretion	Fluid restriction ± dimethylchlortetracycline reduce tumours mass by radiotherapy
Acute Cushing's syndrome	Metyrapone: reduce tumour mass by radiotherapy
Hypercalcaemia	Prednisolone
Gynaecomastia	Tamoxifen

vincristine and methotrexate, of which various combinations have been studied. Chemotherapy of small cell lung cancer is a complex and rapidly changing field in which important advances are being made. We believe that such chemotherapy should, wherever possible, be prescribed and supervised by a physician or oncologist experienced in such therapy. Unskilled use of these powerful drugs may increase the distress of patients without influencing the course of their disease.

Superior vena caval obstruction
Superior vena caval obstruction is usually caused by bronchial carcinoma but may result from lymphoma, mediastinitis or other non-malignant conditions of the mediastinum. In the past it was recommended that superior vena caval obstruction should be regarded as an emergency and that treatment, for presumed bronchial carcinoma, should be started without delaying to confirm the diagnosis. Such patients usually received radiotherapy or chemotherapy and the correct diagnosis was often not established subsequently. It is now known that superior vena caval obstruction in itself carries no threat to life and the authors favour bronchoscopy, mediastinoscopy or mediastinotomy to establish the cause. These carry no additional risk in such patients when performed by experienced operators. Treatment is then based upon the known cause of venous obstruction.

OTHER TUMOURS OF LUNG

Broncho-alveolar ('alveolar cell') carcinoma

This is an adenocarcinoma whose clinical and radiological features differ from the commoner bronchial adenocarcinoma. As the tumour arises in the parenchyma rather than the bronchus obstruction of the bronchus is unusual. The tumour is detected either by finding a localised peripheral opacity or, by cough and breathlessness leading to discovery of one or more areas of consolidation, or multiple nodules on chest X-ray. Tumour may be confined to one lobe but is often more widespread. Extra-thoracic metastases are uncommon.

Diagnosis is often delayed for lung shadows are often wrongly attributed to infection. Adenocarcinoma cells of an unusual type may be identifiable in sputum. Bronchoscopy is often normal but transbronchial biopsy or percutaneous biopsy may yield the diagnosis.

Unless a localised tumour can be removed surgically there is no curative treatment. Breathlessness may be distressing and some patients produce large amounts of mucoid sputum.

Intrathoracic lymphoma

Primary lymphoma of the lung is a rarity, diagnosed only after biopsy or resection. Hodgkin's disease or non-Hodgkin's lymphoma commonly cause enlargment of mediastinal or hilar lymph nodes. Lung involvement is common as the disease progresses but is rarely seen without radiographically obvious enlargement of lymph nodes.

Lymphoma is an uncommon but important cause of pleural effusion.

Pulmonary metastases

These may arise from almost any primary site and are usually multiple when first detected. Lymphatic spread (lymphangitis carcinomatosa) causes linear shadows in the lungs usually with enlarged hilar lymph nodes. Solitary metastases may be difficult to distinguish from primary tumours of the lung.

Identification of the primary source is rarely of clinical value unless:

1. specific chemotherapy is available – e.g. for carcinoma of breast, prostate or thyroid or for testicular tumours
2. resection of a single metastasis or, conceivably, of multiple metastases would be considered (e.g. renal carcinoma, osteogenic sarcoma).

Otherwise a search for a primary tumour is fruitless, time consuming and expensive. Occasionally metastases, especially from breast, kidney or testes, may develop in the bronchial wall causing obstruction and presenting with symptoms, signs and bronchoscopic appearances resembling primary bronchial carcinoma.

Bronchial adenoma

Although the name suggests that these are benign it is better to consider them as tumours of low grade malignancy. Various pathological types are recognised. Symptoms usually result from obstruction of a bronchus and may resemble those of carcinoma. The carcinoid syndrome of flushing, diarrhoea and wheezy breathlessness is rare.

Recurrent haemoptysis, recurrent pneumonia, localised wheeze or lobar collapse will suggest bronchial adenoma if occurring in a young person or a non-smoker. The tumour is usually seen at bronchoscopy but diagnosis from bronchoscopic biopsy may be very difficult and biopsy is said on occasion to cause heavy bleeding. Treatment is surgical either by local resection or lobectomy.

Tumours of the pleura

Most pleural tumours are metastatic and cause pleural effusion (see Chapter 27. It is of benefit to identify the primary site only if this may lead to useful treatment (e.g. chemotherapy for carcinoma of breast or prostate or for small cell lung carcinoma).

Primary malignant mesothelioma

This tumour of the pleura is becoming increasingly common and is usually, but not always, a sequal to exposure to asbestos fibres either at work or casually. The interval between exposure, which may have been only light, and development of the tumour is over 20 years.

Consider malignant mesothelioma, particularly if there has been past exposure to asbestos in a patient with:

— Pleural effusion – either clear or blood stained
— Chest pain, usually aching and not pleuritic
— X-ray which shows, in addition to pleural fluid, pleural masses, widespread pleural thickening or contraction of the hemithorax. These pleural changes may become apparent only after removal of fluid or on computed tomography
— Development of a hard mass in the chest wall after previous aspiration of a pleural effusion for which no cause had been found.

Diagnosis from examination of cells in pleural fluid is difficult and uncertain and pleural biopsy carries the risk of encouraging spread of tumour through the chest wall. If diagnosis is considered essential thoracotomy may be required but also carries the risk of local spread of tumour.

No effective form of treatment is known. In the UK compensation is payable to asbestos workers who develop this tumour.

32. CRYPTOGENIC FIBROSING ALVEOLITIS AND EXTRINSIC ALLERGIC ALVEOLITIS

These two conditions may be very similar in clinical, radiographic and physiological features. Cryptogenic fibrosing alveolitis (CFA) may develop acutely or may be subacute or chronic. Extrinsic allergic alveolitis (EAA) is a hypersensitivity response to inhalation of organic dusts and may likewise be acute, subacute or chronic.

Alveolitis should be suspected in a patient with:

1. Breathlessness on exertion with or without cough but without sputum
2. Bilateral late inspiratory crackles heard usually over the lung bases but sometimes in all areas with or without clubbing of the fingers.

In the acute stages of extrinsic allergic alveolitis fever and weight loss may be so marked that infection is suspected especially as there may be only sparse inspiratory crackles.

Chest X-ray may occasionally be normal in the acute stage, even in patients who are breathless and who have abnormal physical signs. More often there are subtle changes of mid or lower zone haziness with or without tiny nodular opacities. If the changes are more pronounced they may resemble pulmonary oedema or may be mistaken for bilateral pneumonia. In more chronic disease the pattern is of lines and small nodules usually with reduced volume of the lungs. In late CFA the fibrosis is predominantly basal but in chronic EAA it characteristically affects the upper lobes.

Lung function tests show a reduction of vital capacity with proportional reduction of FEV_1, and a low carbon monoxide transfer factor. Arterial oxygen tension may be reduced and CO_2 tension may also be low.

DIFFERENTIAL DIAGNOSIS

Acute illness

In acute illness the following should be considered:

Left ventricular failure and pulmonary oedema
This is often the erroneous diagnosis first made in patients with alveolitis.
If the patient has had no chest pain, has no abnormality on auscultation
of the heart, has a normal blood pressure, has no cardiac enlargement on
X-ray and has a normal ECG the diagnosis of cardiogenic pulmonary
oedema is very unlikely. Other causes of pulmonary oedema such as
postoperative overhydration, inhalation of noxious gases, or the various
types of 'shock lung' should be suspected or discounted from the history.

Infection
Widespread bilateral pneumonia due to virus, mycoplasma or bacterial
infection is usually associated with fever and severe breathlessness.
Miliary tuberculosis may produce widespread nodular shadowing but
extensive inspiratory crackles are rarely heard and breathlessness is not
severe. Pneumonia due to pneumocystis carinii may be clinically and
radiographically very similar to acute alveolitis but occurs almost
invariably in patients with known immune deficiencies.

Malignancy
Widespread metastases involving the pulmonary lymphatics may produce
very similar symptoms which are usually subacute but may develop
rapidly. The patient may be known to have had a primary tumour
(usually of breast, pancreas or stomach). Numerous line shadows of lobar
septa or of distended or obstructed lymphatics are usually seen and will
provide a clue to the diagnosis.

Pulmonary eosinophilia
The radiographic changes are usually quite different from those of acute
alveolitis with patchy areas of consolidation, often in the periphery of the
lung. The diagnosis will be suggested by a marked blood eosinophilia.

Drug reactions (see Chapter 35)

Subacute or chronic illness

Inorganic dust diseases (see Chapter 36)
A history of occupational exposure to coal dust, silica or asbestos will be
obtained if sought. Except in asbestosis inspiratory crackles are not
usually heard.

Bronchiectasis (see Chapter 22)
With extensive bilateral bronchiectasis there will nearly always be a
history of long standing cough, usually with purulent sputum. Clubbing of
the fingers and inspiratory crackles are often present.

Sarcoidosis (see Chapter 33)
In the earlier stages of sarcoidosis X-ray changes are usually
unaccompanied by abnormal signs and breathlessness is absent or slight.
In the late fibrotic stage differentiation between the upper zone fibrosis of
sarcoid and of allergic alveolitis may be very difficult or impossible.

Cryptogenic or allergic alveolitis?

Having considered alternative diagnoses, if alveolitis seems likely, the
following factors should also be considered.

— *Has there been any exposure to organic dusts* known to cause
alveolitis? The commonest domestic hazard in the UK is
inhalation of antigen from pet budgerigars, canaries or from
racing pigeons (bird fancier's lung). Many occupational causes
have been recognised (see Chapter 36), the commonest
probably being Farmers' lung. Most organic dusts may produce
either an acute illness with fever and 'flu like' symptoms or a
subacute or chronic illness with progressive breathlessness. The
acute illness may occur repeatedly and be wrongly labelled 'flu',
bronchitis or pneumonia and awareness of this condition and
careful questioning are needed to discover a time relationship
to inhalation of organic dusts
— *Is there clubbing of the fingers?* Clubbing is present in the
majority of patients with subacute or chronic cryptogenic
fibrosing alveolitis but is much less common in extrinsic
allergic alveolitis
— *Are there joint symptoms?* Cryptogenic fibrosing alveolitis
may be associated with rheumatoid arthritis but many other
patients have transient arthralgia which does not conform to
the criteria of rheumatoid arthritis
— *Are there features to suggest a connective tissue disorder?*
Raynaud's phenomenon with or without skin changes will
suggest systemic sclerosis. The skin and muscle changes of
dermatomyositis may be associated with cryptogenic fibrosing
alveolitis.

Chest X-ray
In the chronic stages lower zone shadowing favours CFA, upper zone
changes favour EAA.

Further investigations

Peripheral blood count
A neutrophil leucocytosis may occur in the acute stage of extrinsic
allergic alveolitis. There is no eosinophilia. The sedimentation rate is
usually raised but this is of no particular diagnostic value.

Rheumatoid factor and anti-nuclear factor
Either anti-nuclear factor or rheumatoid factor is present in the blood of
about two thirds of patients with cryptogenic fibrosing alveolitis although

there may be no other features of rheumatoid disease or systemic lupus erythematosis.

Circulating precipitins
Precipitins may be detected in the blood against the antigen causing extrinsic allergic alveolitis, such as avian proteins (bird fancier's lung), or antigens of either *Micropolyspora faeni* or *Thermoactinomyces vulgaris* (Farmers' lung). With the exception of these two relatively common causes of extrinsic allergic alveolitis the search for precipitins can proceed only when a likely causative substance has been identified. Antibodies may, however, develop in those exposed to the same environment but who do not have lung disease. Therefore detection of precipitins cannot be regarded as proof of a diagnosis of EAA, but merely as useful supporting evidence.

Skin tests
These are usually of no value in diagnosis of EAA because satisfactory antigens are not available. Patients with bird fancier's lung may, however, develop immediate followed by delayed reactions to intradermal injection of avian serum.

Biopsy of the lung
In a patient with typical clinical, radiographic and laboratory features of either cryptogenic fibrosing alveolitis or extrinsic alveolitis, it may be considered that confirmation of the diagnosis by lung biopsy is unnecessary. Often, however, some doubt remains and lung biopsy, in addition to attempting to confirm the diagnosis, is necessary to exclude other conditions the treatment of which may be very different. If the main purpose of biopsy is to exclude or considerably reduce the likelihood of conditions such as disseminated malignancy, miliary tuberculosis, sarcoidosis, alveolar proteinosis or pneumocystis infection, transbronchial biopsies through the fibreoptic bronchoscope (see Chapter 10) may provide sufficient tissue. An alternative is trephine drill biopsy (see Chapter 11). The more fibrotic the lung the lower the likelihood of obtaining a useful transbronchial biopsy. If transbronchial biopsy does not give the necessary information open biopsy is required. The finding of granulomas in lung tissue is much in favour of extrinsic allergic alveolitis rather than cryptogenic fibrosing alveolitis (but there are, of course, many other causes of pulmonary granulomas). It is important that the mere presence of fibrosis in a small lung biopsy is not accepted uncritically as proof of CFA for many other pathological processes may lead to fibrosis.

If it is thought necessary to assess the extent and type of inflammation and fibrosis in a patient with possible or definite CFA the patchy distribution and the variable histological picture makes small biopsies inadequate and an open surgical biopsy (or possibly a trephine or cutting needle biopsy) will be necessary.

Alveolar lavage
The technique of broncho-alveolar lavage during fibreoptic bronchoscopy is still undergoing assessment but may well prove to be of value in distinguishing between some of the causes of diffuse lung shadowing.

Treatment

Extrinsic allergic alveolitis in its acute stages may resolve after complete removal of the causative agent, but if the patient is very breathless or ill oral corticosteroids will speed recovery. Interestingly the carbon monoxide gas transfer factor may remain low even after apparently complete clinical and radiographic recovery. The patient who is breathless with subacute or chronic extrinsic allergic alveolitis will probably require oral corticosteroids.

Acute cryptogenic fibrosing alveolitis may respond rapidly to high doses of oral corticosteroids (40–60 mg prednisolone daily). Patients with more chronic disease may improve on these doses and subsequently be treated with lower doses. Patients who have responded to high doses of corticosteroids but who develop severe side effects at the dose required to maintain control of disease may benefit from adding cyclophosphamide or azothiaprine.

In order to prescribe the lowest effective doses to control the disease, the response to therapy in both CFA and EAA must be carefully monitored by serial good quality chest radiographs and tests of lung function. Repeated alveolar lavage may prove to be a good measure of continued disease activity as a guide to therapy.

33. SARCOIDOSIS

Sarcoidosis is a granulomatous disease characterised by non-caseating granulomas in many organs, especially the lungs, lymph nodes and skin. It should be considered in a patient with one or more of these features:

Non-pulmonary

— Erythema nodosum
— Febrile arthralgia
— Uveitis
— Skin nodules, or plaques or lupus pernio
— Hypercalcaemia

Pulmonary

— Breathlessness (with certain abnormalities on chest X-ray)
— Certain abnormalities on chest X-ray without respiratory symptoms

Pulmonary sarcoidosis is often discovered when a symptom-free person has a chest X-ray. The absence or slightness of symptoms and physical signs with widespread lung shadowing or with enlargement of hilar lymph nodes in itself suggests the possibility of sarcoidosis.

Diagnosis

Diagnosis is usually first considered from a combination of clinical and radiological features.

— *Erythema nodosum with bilateral hilar node enlargement* in a previously healthy young white adult is very likely to be due to sarcoidosis and this diagnosis can usually be accepted without further investigation in parts of the world where systemic mycoses which produce similar features are not endemic

— *Intrathoracic lymph node enlargement* alone. Bilateral hilar node enlargement often with enlarged paratracheal nodes in the absence of symptoms is usually due to sarcoidosis in the UK. Asymmetrical enlargement of paratracheal or hilar nodes, or unilateral hilar node enlargement, raises the question of lymphoma

— *Lymph node enlargement plus lung changes.* Small pulmonary nodules in the mid and upper zones together with bilateral hilar node enlargement strongly suggests sarcoidosis. Such patients are usually well and the disparity between the abnormal chest X-ray and the lack of symptoms and physical signs favours a diagnosis of sarcoid. Lymphoma or disseminated malignancy very rarely produce a similar appearance

— *Lung changes alone:*
   a. Pulmonary nodules without enlargement of lymph nodes. There are many possible causes (see Chapter 38) and further evidence is required to substantiate the diagnosis
   b. Fibrotic changes in the lungs may occur with or without pulmonary nodules and usually take the form of ill defined linear shadows in the mid and upper zones with loss of volume. Cavitation is occasionally seen.

Further investigation

— *ESR and plasma protein* changes are entirely non-specific and of little diagnostic value
— *Tuberculin skin test* is of little practical value in diagnosis as negative tuberculin tests, though frequent in sarcoidosis, are now so common in most populations. Conversion of a previously positive test to negative may occur in sarcoidosis but also in other conditions such as lymphoma. Conversely the tuberculin test may revert to positive during steroid treatment of sarcoidosis
— *X-ray of hands* is not a useful routine investigation as bone lesions are very rare in the absence of skin changes in the hands
— *Serum calcium* measurement is not a rewarding routine test for diagnosis, as hypercalcaemia is rare in the initial stages of sarcoidosis. Hypercalcaemia in sarcoidosis is of such importance however that serum calcium should be measured once a diagnosis of sarcoidosis has been made
— *Serum angiotensin converting enzyme* (ACE) may be elevated in patients with sarcoidosis as compared with normal controls but the clinical value in diagnosis is uncertain, because many patients with sarcoidosis have normal levels and high levels may occur in other conditions which produce pulmonary changes. Changing levels may reflect the activity of the sarcoid process and have been used to assess the response to treatment.
— *Tissue biopsies.* The diagnosis of sarcoidosis is supported by finding non-caseating granulomas in biopsy tissue. Many different tissues may be biopsied:
   a. *Palpable peripheral lymph nodes.* Beware of drawing conclusions from the presence of granulomas in peripheral

nodes as appearances resembling sarcoid may be seen in nodes draining malignant conditions. Biopsy of the scalene fat pad has been outmoded by the greater availability of bronchial and lung biopsy

b. *Mediastinal lymph nodes* can be biopsied at mediastinoscopy or anterior mediastinotomy

c. *Conjunctiva.* Typical histological changes can be found in biopsy of follicles in the lower fornix of the conjunctiva

d. *Skin lesions.* Biopsies of plaques or nodules, if present, may confirm the diagnosis of sarcoidosis

e. *Liver* biopsy was widely used before the advent of transbronchial lung biopsy but, though giving a high yield in sarcoidosis, is of limited value because of the lack of specificity of non-caseating liver granulomas

f. *Biopsy of the lung.* Biopsy of the bronchial mucosa or lung at fibreoptic bronchoscopy yields typical histological changes in about 80% of patients with bilateral hilar node enlargement alone or with pulmonary nodules. The yield is much smaller when fibrosis has developed.

At bronchoscopy the mucosa may appear normal or may have an appearance resembling cobblestones but typical granulomas may be found in both normal and abnormal mucosa. Lung tissue may be histologically abnormal even without pulmonary shadowing i.e. in a patient with enlarged hilar nodes alone. It is our policy to attempt biopsy of both bronchial mucosa and lung if a diagnosis of sarcoidosis is suspected

g. *The Kveim test.* Intradermal injection of suspension of sarcoid spleen produces a local reaction containing epitheliod cell tubercles.

Technique: 0.1 ml of test suspension is injected intradermally into the volar surface of the forearm. The suspension should be shaken before being taken into the syringe. The site of injection must be marked by pricking the skin on both sides of the injection through a drop of sterile Indian ink. A mild local erythema may develop rapidly but subsides within a few days and a papule often develops in the succeeding weeks. The presence of such a papule is not in itself sufficient evidence of a positive Kveim reaction nor does the absence of a visible or palpable nodule indicate a negative result. Biopsy of the injection site is necessary whether or not a papule can be felt. Biopsy is best performed at 5 to 6 weeks after injection by skin punch biopsy of the exact site of injection.

Histological interpretation of the biopsy is not without difficulty and observer variation. A typical positive reaction containing epithelioid cell tubercles may be accepted as confirming the diagnosis if other features, clinical or radiographic, are consistent with the diagnosis of sarcoidosis. A normal biopsy does not exclude the diagnosis and may be found in one third of patients in the early stages of sarcoidosis and two thirds with chronic sarcoidosis. Positive Kveim reactions may occasionally be obtained in patients with Crohn's disease, ulcerative colitis, coeliac disease and tuberculous lymphadenitis. Because of the unavoidable delay before obtaining a result and because of problems of interpretation of the findings the Kveim test is less widely used for diagnosis of sarcoidosis now that biopsy of lung and bronchial mucosa are more readily available.

— *Tests of lung function.* There are no specific or diagnostic features. Patients with bilateral hilar node enlargement usually have normal spirometry and tests of gas transfer, and even some of those with extensive pulmonary mottling also give normal results in these tests. The commonest abnormality in patients with widespread lung shadowing is reduction of vital capacity and lung volumes without evidence of airflow obstruction but with reduced carbon monoxide transfer factor. These changes worsen as pulmonary fibrosis develops. Occasional patients show an obstructive picture which should raise the possibility of sarcoid bronchostenosis or of coexistent asthma. Tests of lung function are more valuable to assess the course and response to treatment than as a guide to intial diagnosis.

Natural history, course and prognosis

Conflicting opinions about the natural history and prognosis of pulmonary sarcoidosis (and therefore about treatment) reflect differences in the behaviour of the disease in different races and the difficulties of carrying out satisfactory long-term studies.

In general however erythema nodosum with bilateral hilar node enlargement carries a very good prognosis. In the UK, 90% of more of such patients recover to a normal chest X-ray without treatment although this may take several years. The prognosis of patients with pulmonary nodules is less certain for a proportion progress to fibrosis. However the radiographic and physiological abnormalities frequently improve spontaneously making the assessment of response to treatment very difficult.

Pulmonary fibrosis develops in fewer than 5% of all patients with intrathoracic sarcoidosis.

The small pulmonary nodules may disappear while linear shadowing and loss of volume of the mid and especially the upper zones increases, sometimes with cavitation. By this time the patient is usually breathless on exertion with markedly reduced vital capacity and CO transfer factor. Hypoxaemia may develop with eventual respiratory failure and right heart failure. Pneumothorax is an occasional complication of pulmonary fibrosis and colonisation of cavities with aspergillus fumigatus may lead to a mycetoma which can cause severe haemoptysis.

Management

Erythema nodosum with bilateral hilar node enlargement
Many such patients have no symptoms once the erythema nodosum has subsided and require no treatment. Fever and other systemic symptoms usually respond to salicylates or non-steroidal anti-inflammatory drugs but occasional patients are ill enough to require a short course of oral steroids.

Patients with pulmonary nodules
There is no consensus on the management of this group of patients. It is our policy to treat with oral corticosteroids if patients become breathless, develop deterioration of lung function tests, if diffuse lung changes worsen on serial X-rays or if radiological changes of fibrosis develop. There are others however who treat with corticosteroids if radiographic shadowing persists after an observation period which varies between 6 months and 2 years.

If corticosteroids are to be given it is usual to start with a dose of at least 30 mg of prednisolone daily. This dose is subsequently reduced, guided by changes in X-ray and lung function tests. Other methods of assessing response to treatment such as serial measurements of angiotensin converting enzyme, gallium lung scans or bronchoalveolar lavage are currently under investigation. It is important to recognise that patients who require corticosteroids for treatment of sarcoidosis may continue to need these drugs for a very long time. Whether oral corticosteroids merely suppress the radiographic features or prevent ultimate fibrosis is not known.

Extra thoracic sarcoidosis
Oral steroid therapy is necessary if there is involvement of the heart or central nervous system or development of hypercalcaemia and for some types of eye involvement. If eye symptoms develop the importance of seeking expert advice cannot be over-emphasised for ocular sarcoidosis can lead to blindness.

Sarcoidosis involving the heart is probably more common than is generally recognised. Many patients with cardiac sarcoid have no readily detected evidence of disease elsewhere but the development of dysrhythmias in a patient known to have sarcoidosis should be assumed to be the result of cardiac involvement and the risk of fatal arrythmia is such that oral steroid treatment should be considered even in the absence of disease elsewhere.

34. CHEST INJURIES

Chest injuries may result in rapid impairment of respiration and of circulation. They are frequently associated with major trauma to other parts of the body which makes for difficulty in determining priorities for treatment. However, external haemorrhage is the only condition which takes precedence over restoration of circulation and respiration.

INITIAL ASSESSMENT AND MANAGEMENT

Because of the urgency of the situation, diagnosis and treatment must proceed simultaneously.

1. Is the patient breathing? If not, start artificial respiration with a tightly applied face mask and bag to which an oxygen supply should be connected as soon as possible. Summon an anaesthetist urgently to insert an endotracheal tube

2. Is there respiratory distress, stridor, cyanosis or evidence of choking? These features suggest respiratory obstruction, which may be due to a foreign body, inhaled vomit or inhaled blood. Pass a finger into the back of the pharynx to search for and remove any foreign body, and then suck out the pharynx and larynx, if possible with the aid of a laryngoscope. If respiratory obstruction persists send for an anaesthetist, or a thoracic surgeon to aspirate the bronchial tree with a rigid bronchoscope (the fibreoptic bronchoscope is far less satisfactory for this purpose). Remember that obstruction can often be overcome by ventilation with oxygen under pressure. To relieve obstruction caused by the tongue falling back in the unconscious patient pull the angles of the jaw firmly upwards. Before any movement or manipulation of the patient consider the possibility of a fracture of the cervical spine.

3. Look for a tension pneumothorax. This is suggested by unequal movement of the two sides of the chest. One side may be immobile and in young patients bulging of the intercostal spaces may be seen on the affected side. The

most reliable sign is deviation of the trachea to the opposite side. Palpate the trachea at the level of the suprasternal notch to elicit this sign.

If you are sure that the patient has a tension pneumothorax insert a large bore needle in the second intercostal space in the mid-clavicular line. If the diagnosis is correct you will hear a hiss as the air escapes. Leave the needle in situ and obtain a chest radiograph immediately. Do not waste time on detailed auscultation of the chest. In only a few seconds you can discover whether there are breath sounds on one side and none on the other, but surgical emphysema or the patient's movements may render this examination useless.

4. Is the patient suffering from shock or internal haemorrhage, manifested by a rapid pulse, low or unrecordable blood pressure and collapsed veins? If so an intravenous infusion of a colloid solution such as haemaccel should be set up without delay. Do not waste time trying to cannulate collapsed veins, but send for someone experienced in inserting a central venous line, and proceed to a venous cut-down only if their arrival is likely to be delayed. As soon as a vein has been entered blood should be obtained for cross-matching

5. External bleeding from the chest should be controlled by pressure. An open chest wound is covered with a sterile dressing

6. Is there a weapon or embedded object protruding from the chest? In spite of the temptation to remove it, leave it untouched. It may be a sealing a hole in the heart or one of the great vessels

7. Is there a flail segment of the chest wall which is being sucked in with each inspiration? If the area is extensive and the patient is cyanosed and dyspnoeic, endotracheal intubation and artificial ventilation is necessary. However in many cases relief of respiratory obstruction and of pain will result in diminution or disappearance of the paradoxical movement

8. Is the patient in pain? If so give repeated small doses of intravenous omnopon, about 3 mg at a time for an adult. The dose can be titrated against the pain and since the effect is short-lived the assessment of head and abdominal injuries is not compromised

9. Is there venous congestion in the neck? This may be the result of mediastinal haemorrhage (for example from a ruptured aorta,) choking, previous over-transfusion or cardiac tamponade

10. Is there surgical emphysema in the neck? If this has

developed early it suggests rupture of the trachea or of a main bronchus

11. Has the patient coughed up blood? This is to be expected if there is extensive laceration of the face, or pharyngeal haemorrhage from a fracture of the base of the skull. In the absence of these conditions tracheal or bronchial rupture should be suspected.

While this emergency assessment and treatment is being carried out, make arrangements for a chest radiograph to be obtained as soon as possible.

FURTHER MANAGEMENT

Pneumothorax

A suspected pneumothorax should be dealt with immediately by insertion of a needle or flexible intravenous cannula into the second intercostal space as previously described. If the radiograph confirms a pneumothorax a tube should be inserted into the pleural space (see Chapter 41).

'Prophylactic' tube insertion
Some authorities consider that if the patient is to be ventilated mechanically, especially when it is necessary to use high inflation pressures, tubes should be inserted into both pleural cavities to deal with a tension pneumothorax which may develop. If this policy, which involves insertion of a tube into a normal pleural space, is to be followed it is essential that the method of tube insertion described in Chapter 41 is carried out. Without careful dissection down to the pleural space there is a high probability that the tube will enter or damage the lung.

Fractures of the thoracic skeleton

Chest wall injuries may result in various patterns of fractured ribs and fractures of the sternum, but these fractures are not often visible on the initial chest radiograph. Remember that in the elderly chronic bronchitic a single rib fracture may have serious effects on respiratory function. A common injury is the fracture of several adjacent ribs at their anterior and posterior ends, which may give rise to a lateral flail segment. Transverse fracture of the sternum is often accompanied by bilateral fractures of the anterior ends of several ribs or costal cartilages resulting in an anterior flail chest.

Pain relief

If adequate pain relief is not provided the patient breathes shallowly and will not cough. As a result he will become dyspnoeic and cyanosed from sputum retention and lobar collapse, thus converting a relatively harmless condition to a serious and even life-threatening one. Prophylaxis is by adequate pain relief. Intermittent intravenous omnopon in doses of 3 mg at a time is the ideal first aid treatment. Later analgesia can be provided by continuous intravenous omnopon at a rate of 1–8 mg per hour, intercostal blocks with Marcaine or by paravertebral or epidural block. There is no danger of respiratory depression so long as the recommended doses are not exceeded, unless the patient has severe chronic bronchitis, a fact which may not be recognised unless the patient or relatives are specifically questioned on this point.

Flail chest

If the chest wall is extensively disrupted on both sides immediate artificial ventilation via an endotracheal tube is essential. However, in the majority of patients with flail chest the paradoxical movement is of little importance. The so called pendulum movement of air between the two lungs, which was thought to result from this condition, has in fact never been demonstrated. The flail segment in itself does not require any treatment unless it appears that gross chest deformity will result. In that case a thoracic surgeon should be called in early because internal fixation is often the best treatment.

The paradoxical movement of a flail chest is exaggerated by high intrapleural negative pressures caused by unrelieved pain, by atelectasis from sputum retention or by airflow obstruction. These should be managed by adequate analgesia, by physiotherapy and by energetic medical treatment of airflow obstruction.

Blood gases

No mention has been made of the measurement of blood gases so far, since in the early stages of management these are unimportant compared with a clinical assessment of the adequacy of ventilation. In the ventilated patient the blood gases should be measured regularly so that the ventilator can be appropriately adjusted.

In patients breathing spontaneously, especially if they are young and fit, an arterial partial pressure of oxygen of about 8 kPa and of CO_2 of 7–8 kPa are quite acceptable. Many neurosurgeons would be prepared to accept these figures even in the presence of head injury. Remember that if the P_{O_2} is low and the P_{CO_2} not grossly raised the appropriate treatment is oxygen at high concentration. It is quite safe to give oxygen freely to these patients for the first 24 hours. The administration of only 28% or 35% oxygen to a severely hypoxic patient is a common and serious error.

Artificial ventilation

Artificial ventilation is clearly necessary immediately if the patient is not
breathing, is deeply cyanosed or if there is extensive haemorrhage around
or disruption of the face and trachea. It should however be discontinued
as soon as possible. If patients with chest injuries are ventilated
artificially for more than 1 or 2 days, for example in cases of instability of
the chest wall, it is usually found that the treatment must be continued
for 2–3 weeks. A tracheostomy will then be required which leaves the
patient at a high risk of infection of the lungs with gram-negative
organisms, and consequent gram-negative septicaemia.

Indications for tracheostomy

— Prolonged artificial ventilation
— Prolonged unconciousness associated with a severe chest
  injury, to facilitate aspiration of tracheobronchial secretions
— When bronchoscopy has been necessary on two occasions for
  the removal of secretions. In these patients frequent
  tracheobronchial suction will probably continue to be
  necessary and tracheostomy avoids further bronchoscopies.
  'Mini-tracheostomy' has recently been recommended
  in this situation.

Pulmonary contusion

In patients with chest trauma much of the respiratory difficulty is due
more to the accompanying pulmonary contusion than to the chest wall
damage. This contusion is usually but not always visible on the initial
chest X-ray but becomes obvious as diffuse areas of opacification develop
12 or more hours later. In the contused areas the capillaries become
permeable to crystalloids, infusion of which rapidly produces pulmonary
oedema. Crystalloid fluids are potentially harmful to patients with chest
injury. On the other hand administration of diuretics leads to
improvement in blood gases before pulmonary infiltrates are visible. As
far as possible therefore intravenous crystalloid fluids for resuscitation
should be limited to 1 l, and subsequently fluid should be given at a rate
no greater than 50 ml per hour. The patient should also receive 40 mg
frusemide daily. Moreover, the incidence of pulmonary infection is
reduced if the lungs are kept dry. Blood or colloidal solutions should be
given to maintain an adequate circulatory volume if haemorrhage is
severe.

Intrapleural bleeding

1. If the patient is exsanguinating and the site of bleeding can
   be localised to one side of the chest, immediate operation is
   essential

2. Major or continued haemorrhage. Major haemorrhage is defined as the drainage of 1 l or more of blood through a chest drain inserted into the pleural cavity. Continued haemorrhage is bleeding of the order of 200 ml per hour for more than 4 hours. In these two circumstances thoracotomy should be performed. A major bleeding source will nearly always be encountered.

If a haemothorax is not treated early the blood will clot. A small clotted haemothorax will resolve spontaneously but a large one occupying more than one third of the pleural cavity will result in a fibrothorax and therefore thoracotomy for decortication may eventually be required.

Chest X-rays

Supine chest X-rays provide a limited amount of information compared with films taken in the erect position. If there is any doubt about the interpretation of the chest X-ray a second film should be obtained whenever possible with the patient upright. This can be achieved in most patients even when there is persistent hypotension by the following method:

One nurse reads the blood pressure while the X-ray tube is placed in position and the film cassette is placed beneath the patient. 2 mg of metaraminol is given intravenously and the blood pressure is called out. As it begins to rise several helpers lift the patient and cassette into the upright position and the exposure is made.

Before this procedure, and indeed before laryngoscopy, bronchoscopy or any other movement of the patient, every effort must be made to exclude a fracture of the cervical spine. Decubitus films or a lateral film with a horizontal beam are good alternative methods of looking for a pneumothorax.

Penetrating lung wounds

These rarely require thoracotomy although pleural intubation may be necessary for the treatment of a pneumothorax or haemothorax.

Embedded instruments and objects

These must not be disturbed. The patient is taken to the operating theatre and an appropriate thoracotomy carried out so as to expose the likely mediastinal structures involved. The great vessels are mobilised and snared and if necessary cardiopulmonary bypass instituted. When complete control of the circulation has been obtained the foreign body is removed and an appropriate repair carried out.

Ruptured bronchus

This should be suspected in the presence of the following signs:
— Gross mediastinal emphysema and cervical emphysema
— Bilateral pneumothoraces which leak a large amount of air continuously
— Haemoptysis.

Bronchoscopy should be carried out early. The bronchial tear is not usually visible, but haemorrhage and oedema at the carina or in one or other main bronchus confirms the diagnosis. An immediate thoracotomy and repair of the tear should be carried out. If the diagnosis is missed bronchial stenosis will occur at the site of the tear leading to complete collapse of the lung, and the degree of fibrosis then surrounding the bronchus and main pulmonary artery makes repair impossible so that a pneumonectomy is often inevitable.

Ruptured diaphragm

This occurs more commonly on the left and the diagnosis is frequently missed. On the erect chest radiograph the outline of the distended stomach commonly appears as an curved line in the lower half of the left hemithorax. The appearance may easily be misinterpreted as a high diaphragm with a distended stomach beneath it or even as a pneumothorax.

The diagnosis can be confirmed by an antero-posterior chest radiograph with the patient in the lateral decubitus position which will show two fluid levels, one above and one below the diaphragm, outlining the diaphragm between them. A barium swallow is necessary only if the diagnosis remains in doubt. The obstructed distended stomach in the thorax may sometimes give rise to respiratory difficulty and it may be possible to decompress it before operation by the passage of a nasogastric tube.

The colon and small intestine may sometimes migrate into the thorax alongside the stomach. The characteristic chest radiograph shows a opacified hemithorax with many fluid levels. Thoracotomy is necessary to repair the diaphragm without delay.

Traumatic rupture of the aorta

The occurence of this is usually just below the level of the left subclavian artery. Suspect aortic rupture if there is:
— Raised jugular venous pressure
— Unexplained hypertension
— Widening of the mediastinum on the chest radiograph
— Left haemothorax.

There are many causes of mediastinal widening after a chest injury but it should always be assumed that the cause is a rupture of the aorta and a thoracic surgeon should be consulted immediately. The two ends of the aorta usually part completely, but the haematoma is held in place by the adventitia. This however may rupture at any time, especially if the blood pressure rises. An aortogram is essential to establish the diagnosis. Before any investigation or treatment is carried out an intravenous infusion of sodium nitroprusside should be set up and the systolic blood pressure lowered to about 80 mmHg.

When the diagnosis has been confirmed an immediate left thoracotomy is carried out. The damaged area is replaced by a synthetic graft. While the aorta is clamped the spinal cord and kidneys are protected from ischaemia by a heparin-bonded plastic tube bypass from the ascending to the descending aorta.

Non-penetrating cardiac injuries

Blows to the front of the chest, or anteroposterior compression, may result in temporary dysrhythmias, or damage to the coronary arteries resulting in myocardial infarction. Rupture of any of the heart valves or of the ventricular septum may occur. Haemopericardium can also result leading to cardiac tamponade. A cardiologist should be consulted. Most of these conditions are treated conservatively, but the onset of heart failure may be an indication for detailed investigation. Cardiac tamponade requires immediate surgical relief.

Penetrating wounds of the heart and great vessels

Any penetrating or probably penetrating wounds in the area of the front of the chest between the clavicle and epigastrium, and between the right mid-clavicular line and the left mid-axillary line should be regarded as having penetrated the heart or one of the great vessels. The same applies to any wound in a similar area posteriorly. Immediate exploration is called for irrespective of whether there is any manifestation of cardiac tamponade. The reason for this is that the right-sided chambers of the heart, being low pressure areas, quite frequently stop bleeding for a time. Bleeding may recur as a result of a rise of blood pressure caused by transfusion or by exertion. If cardiac tamponade is followed by cardiac arrest the chances of saving the patient are slight. The policy of immediate exploration is therefore justified even although the operation will occasionally be found to have been unnecessary.

Cardiac tamponade

The cardinal features are a falling blood pressure associated with a raised jugular venous pressure. Transfusion increases the venous pressure without any effect on the arterial pressure. Pulsus paradoxus is difficult to elicit and no time should be wasted on seeking it in these emergency cases.

Oesophageal injury

Penetrating wounds of the thorax on either side of the spine should be regarded as having involved the oesophagus. The diagnosis should be confirmed by barium swallow which is much more useful than oesophagoscopy in this situation. Treatment is by immediate surgical repair.

Conclusion

For the successful management of these patients an anaesthetist should be on hand at the earliest possible moment, and a thoracic surgeon should be called in before complications develop.

35. DRUG INDUCED LUNG DISEASE

It has been estimated that about one in ten of all patients admitted to general medical wards is suffering from an adverse affect of drug therapy. The cause of their illness is frequently not recognised and this is particularly so in patients with drug induced respiratory disease.
Drugs may cause:
— Asthma
— Breathlessness with or without cough
— Pulmonary shadowing
— Pleural effusion (uncommon)
— Intrathoracic lymph node enlargement (uncommon)
— Mediastinal fibrosis (uncommon)

ASTHMA

Previous, but often unrecognised, asthma may be worsened or symptoms may develop for the first time as a result of drug therapy.

Beta blocking agents
All of those currently available may precipitate asthmatic attacks although the 'cardio-selective' preparations may be less likely to do. Severe attacks may follow a single dose and have occurred even after eye drops containing such drugs. Some patients with chronic bronchitis and 'irreversible' airflow obstruction may become more breathless when treated with beta blocking agents.

Analgesics
Aspirin (which is often present unbeknown to patients and doctors in over-the-counter remedies) may produce severe asthma, particularly in patients who have nasal polyps. Many other analgesics including paracetamol, indomethacin, pentazocine and dextropropoxyphene may have the same effect.

Other drugs
Asthma may develop as part of a generalised hypersensitivity reaction (penicillins, radiographic contrast media, iron-dextran infusions, desensitizing injections), due to inhaled drugs (including, very rarely,

those used in the treatment of asthma) or agents used to induce anaesthesia. Tartrazine dyes used as colouring agents for tablets and foods have been implicated as a precipitating factor in asthma.

Recognising the problem

Confirm the diagnosis of asthma
This is straightforward if a bilateral expiratory wheeze is heard but in the absence of wheeze spirometry may confirm airflow obstruction, reversible with inhaled bronchodilators, or if symptoms are intermittent, serial peak flow measurements may show the fluctuations characteristic of asthma (see Chapter 30).

Consider the relationship to therapy
If the possibility of a drug effect has been recognised the time-association of symptoms with starting new drugs may be obvious, or the effect on both symptoms and spirometry of stopping a possibly responsible drug should be assessed. Challenge with the drug under suspicion, even in small doses, may be hazardous and is to be avoided unless absolutely necessary.

Management

If asthma is caused or exacerbated by aspirin or is part of a generalised hypersensitivity reaction the offending drug and any closely related drugs should not be taken again. The patient, his other doctors, and, if need be, close relatives should be told of the risk of severe asthma if the drug is used again and all should be advised to read carefully the small print on the package before taking any proprietary medicines. Hospital records should be clearly marked with a warning. If a beta blocking drug has been responsible every effort should be made to devise an alternative form of treatment for the underlying disease but if this is not possible then one of the more 'cardio-selective' agents may be tolerated especially if taken together with regular inhaled adrenergic bronchodilators. The first few doses of any new beta blocking drug should however be taken under close supervision in hospital.

NON-ASTHMATIC DIFFUSE PULMONARY REACTIONS

An adverse reaction to current or recent drugs should be considered in patients with:
>   — breathlessness without wheeze
>   — dry cough
>   — pulmonary shadowing on X-ray.

It is often difficult or impossible to incriminate a drug with certainty but if in doubt any drug which has the reputation of causing lung damage should be stopped. If improvement follows, a causal relationship is still uncertain but, unless essential, further use of that drug is unwise. The mechanisms of drug-induced lung damage are not always clear and some drugs may produce a range of different types of adverse reaction.

Pulmonary eosinophilia (see also Chapter 37)

Respiratory symptoms may be slight with little more than cough and malaise, or there may be breathlessness, fever and weight loss. A drug-induced condition is suggested by blood eosinophilia and changes on X-ray which may range from patchy segmental opacities to widespread fine nodular shadowing.

Commonly used drugs which may be responsible include
— sulphonamides (by any route including local application)
— sulphasalazine
— chlorpropamide
— imipramine
— mephenesin
— nitrofurantoin.

The patient with pulmonary eosinophilia should if possible stop all oral and local drugs and the drug believed to be responsible should not be taken again.

Diffuse pulmonary reaction without eosinophilia

Several drugs may cause an illness with breathlessness, dry cough, possibly fever, inspiratory crackles on auscultation and widespread pulmonary shadowing on chest X-ray. The mechanisms of lung damage may differ beteween different drugs and respiratory symptoms may develop soon after starting the drug or after several months of therapy. They usually subside with complete radiologial and physiological resolution on stopping the drug which should not be used again.

The more commonly used drugs which may produce this pattern of illness include:
— sulphasalazine
— methotrexate
— procarbazine
— azothiaprine
— chlorambucil
— penicillamine
— nitrofurantoin.

Diffuse pulmonary reaction which may lead to fibrosis

Symptoms and X-ray appearances similar to those described above may progress to lung fibrosis, sometimes even after withdrawal of the drug.

The more commonly used drugs which may be responsible are:
- busulphan
- bleomycin
- cyclophosphamide
- melphelan
- methotrexate
- gold salts
- nitrofurantoin
- amiodarone.

The reaction to some of these drugs, notably bleomycin, seems to be related to total dosage and early changes can sometimes be detected by careful scrutiny of serial chest X-rays or by serial lung function tests which show a fall of vital capacity and of carbon monoxide transfer factor. Pulmonary damage is said to be greater if bleomycin is given together with irradiation of the lungs. The drug under suspicion must be withdrawn but continued deterioration may follow and may not respond to corticosteroids. Fibrosis due to amiodarone may develop long after the drug has been stopped and a careful history of previous as well as present drug usage is essential.

Drug induced lupus syndrome

This may produce a pleural effusion with or without pain, clinical and X-ray features resembling pneumonia or pulmonary infarction, or breathlessness with few abnormal physical signs but with raised diaphragms on chest X-ray. Diagnosis depends on suspicion of systemic lupus and knowledge of the more commonly used drugs which may produce this type of adverse effect:
- procainamide
- phenytoin
- hydrallazine
- isoniazid
- chlorpromazine
- penicillamine.

36. OCCUPATION AND LUNG DISEASE

Occupational factors may cause respiratory disease in various ways:
— Inhalation of mineral dusts which may:
    a. be inert
    b. cause fibrosis of lung (or pleura)
    c. cause granulomas
— Immunological mechanisms (chemicals or organic dusts)
    a. asthma
    b. alveolitis
— Irritant or toxic (gases, fumes, dusts)
    a. high concentrations –
        pulmonary oedema
        acute bronchitis
        asthma
    b. low concentrations –
        chronic bronchitis
        worsening of asthma
— Carcinogens

Some clinical situations in which an occupational cause should be considered are shown in Table 36.1.

Table 36.1 Occupation and lung disease. An occupational cause should be considered in these clinical situations

Clinical and radiological picture	Consider occupational exposure to
Diffuse small round shadows on chest X-ray (with or without breathlessness)	Coal dust, silica, iron, tin, barium
Fibrosing alveolitis picture	Organic dusts (extrinsic allergic alveolitis) Asbestos
Resembling sarcoidosis	Beryllium
Bilateral upper zone fibrosis	Organic dusts (extrinsic allergic alveolitis) Beryllium
Pleural plaques	Asbestos
Bilateral upper zone opacities (with or without breathlessness)	Coal, silica
Asthma of late onset	See Table 36.2.
Pulmonary oedema	Irritant gases and fumes

Occupational disease may be *acute* (and related to present or very recent exposure) such as acute alveolitis, recent asthma, non-cardiac pulmonary oedema; or *chronic* (and related either to long periods of continuing exposure or to past, and maybe forgotten, exposure) such as simple or complicated pneumoconiosis, advanced fibrosis from alveolitis, long standing asthma or malignancy.

The occupational history

Basic occupational history
This should be sought from all patients with respiratory or other disease, even if there is no diagnostic problem.
> — Is the illness related to work factors?
> — Does the illness have implications for future work?

Diagnostic occupational history
This requires questions which will differ depending on the type of condition under investigation, being slanted towards occupational factors which are known to be relevant to that condition. Important questions include the following:

Present job
> — What exactly does the present job entail?
> — What materials or processes are used?
> — What is the intensity and duration of exposure to dusts or fumes?
> — How do symptoms relate in time to hours of work, periods away from work or different activities at work?
> — Are any precautions taken or advised at work?
> — Do others working in the same job have similar symptoms?
> — Have others working in the same job left that employment because of similar symptoms?
> — Any part-time jobs or hobbies outside working hours?

Previous jobs
A complete list should be made, answering the above questions for each.

If it seems that symptoms or other features may be related to a specific substance or process, information or known effects of such exposure should be sought from reference books, or from Units specialising in occupational diseases.

ASTHMA AND OCCUPATION

The diagnosis of asthma is discussed in Chapter 30. The importance, both for the patient and for others in the same job, of recognising an occupational cause was emphasised together with the features of asthma which should raise suspicion of an occupational cause (see p 171).

Occupational factors may influence the development of asthma in various ways:

— Dusts, fumes, chemicals or cold air may act as non-specific 'triggers' of asthma in workers with pre-existing asthma (whether the asthma was previously recognised or not)
— A temporary 'asthmatic state' may be induced by inhalation of certain reactive chemicals such as chlorine
— Hypersensitivity to a substance encountered at work may cause true 'occupational asthma'. Such a substance is truly responsible for inducing the asthmatic state.

The term 'occupational asthma' is usually only applied to the third of the above cases.

Sequence of diagnosis of occupational asthma

1. Diagnosis of asthma (see Chapter 30)
2. Suspicion of a possible occupational cause (Table 36.2)
3. Confirmation of association with occupation
4. Differentiation between specific and non-specific causes
5. Identification of the agent responsible.

Table 36.2 Some commoner causes of occupational asthma

Responsible agent	Occupation
Urinary proteins from small mammals	Workers in animal laboratories (rats, mice etc)
Flour, grain	Food industry, bakers, farmers
Exotic wood dusts	Wood mill workers, carpenters
Solder flux (colophony)	Electronics workers
Isocyanates	Manufacture or heating of polyurethane Printing Manufacture of synthetic paints or of rubber adhesives
Epoxy resins	Adhesives, coatings
Platinum salts	Platinum refinery

To confirm an association with occupation

Although a history of asthma starting after beginning a new job or a new process, or occurring in a job which is known to carry a risk of occupational asthma, suggests an occupational cause, proof is required before a patient can be advised to alter his work or a factory to alter their processes.

Serial measurements of peak flow

The patient borrows a peak flow meter and records the best of three measurements several times every day throughout the waking hours for several weeks. An ideal is peak flow records every 2 hours. This obviously requires willing collaboration of the patient (and also honesty in recording the results).

Look at the records for:
— Any difference between days at work or away from work? (weekends, holidays)
— Any of variation of peak flow?
  a. A fall of PEF during each working shift returns to normal after stopping work
  b. A progressive fall of PEF during the working week, sometimes with delayed recovery so that a progressive fall continues over several weeks. Longer periods away from work than usual weekends are necessary to see any return to normal. (These patients are at particular risk of being labelled 'chronic bronchitis' as there is little apparent variation of peak flow)
  c. Progressive deterioration week after week
  d. Greatest deterioration on the first day back at work after a break

Night-time asthma after daytime exposure at work. Some patterns are characteristic of (but by no means diagnostic of) specific causes of occupational asthma.

Asthma due to hypersensitivity or a non-specific effect of occupation
Non-specific stimuli which provoke asthma in workers with pre-existing asthma (or bronchial hyper-reactivity):
— may trigger an attack on first exposure (which never occurs from allergic hypersensitivity)
— usually cause symptoms within minutes of exposure which subside in 1–2 hours
— cause symptoms in workers who have had previous symptoms (recognised or unrecognised) of asthma and whose symptoms often continue when away from work.

Reactive chemicals which cause a temporary asthmatic state usually cause symptoms after accidental exposure to a high concentration, as after a leakage or spillage. Symptoms improve over days or weeks and do not recur on exposure to concentrations of the same substance which other workers can tolerate without symptoms.

Hypersensitivity reactions are recognised from the various patterns of peak flow described above.

Identification of the responsible agent

Skin tests
Prick tests (see Chapter 14) with specific industrial allergens may be positive in patients with some types of occupational asthma but are not applicable to others. Skin responses may, however, reflect only sensitisation which is probably, but not necessarily, the cause of the asthma.

Serological tests
Specific serum IgE antibodies may be present against some occupational allergens but, like positive skin tests, only indicate sensitisation and are not proof of a causal association with asthma.

Bronchial provocation (challenge) tests
Rarely inhalation of a suspected agent is justifiable to:
- — confirm the diagnosis of occupational asthma if other tests have been inconclusive
- — identify a previously unrecognised cause of asthma.

These tests carry the risk of precipitating severe asthma and should be carried out only by those experienced in the techniques and interpretation and under conditions where an early or delayed asthmatic attack can be treated.

Non-specific bronchial provocation (challenge) tests (see p 159)
Most occupational asthma is associated with development of bronchial hyper-reactivity which can be detected by provocation with histamine (see Chapter 30). This hyper-reactivity then usually declines on avoidance of the responsible agent. This test can be used to identify workers who are at greatest risk while working in occupations which carry a known risk of occupational asthma.

Management and prognosis

Most workers with proven occupational asthma are best advised to seek alternative work or to seek another job in a different area of the factory. If this is not practicable conventional treatment of asthma with prophylactic inhaled steroids or cromoglycate and bronchodilator drugs (see Chapter 30) may be effective but careful observation with serial tests of lung function is essential to identify any deterioration as soon as possible.

Most, but not quite all, workers with occupational asthma lose their symptoms when no longer exposed to the specific cause.

Compensation

In the UK workers suffering from some types of occupational asthma are eligible for statutory compensation. The list of prescribed causes is frequently reviewed and the current position can be discovered from official publications. The more commonly encountered prescribed causes include isocyanates, some hardening agents, soldering flux resins, laboratory animals, flour or grain dust. Claims are made by the patient via the local offices of the Department of Health and Social Security.

MINERAL DUST PNEUMOCONIOSIS

Inert dusts

Inert dusts (such as metallic iron or iron oxide, tin or barium) produce dense nodular opacities, seen on chest X-ray, which cause no lung damage or loss of function.

Coal workers pneumoconiosis

The risk of developing coal workers pneumoconiosis is related to the level and duration of exposure to respirable coal dust. 'Simple pneumoconiosis' is a radiological (or pathological) diagnosis. Small 2–5 mm nodules are seen in both lungs, occasionally with larger 10 mm nodules, but without impairment of lung function. Hence if a coal worker with simple pneumoconiosis has respiratory symptoms these must be from some other cause (often chronic bronchitis and emphysema from cigarette smoking).

'Complicated pneumoconiosis' (massive fibrosis) develops in some coal workers with simple pneumoconiosis who remain exposed to coal dust. Large areas of pulmonary fibrosis develop and are seen on X-ray as masses, usually initially in the upper lobes, which in time are accompanied by bullous emphysema. There is breathlessness with airflow obstruction and other features of emphysema. Cor pulmonale or respiratory failure may develop.

Caplan's syndrome of 1 to 4 cm nodules in the lungs of coal workers who have rheumatoid arthritis or rheumatoid factor in the serum may cause no symptoms. The lesions may cavitate and must be distinguished from other causes of pulmonary nodules.

Treatment

Simple pneumoconiosis needs no treatment other than removal from further exposure to coal dust. Apart from treatment for symptoms of emphysema and its complications there is no specific therapy for the massive fibrosis of complicated pneumoconiosis. Coal workers pneumoconiosis is not associated with an increased risk of tuberculosis or cancer.

Silicosis

This results from prolonged occupational inhalation of silica-containing dusts in such jobs as foundry work, lens grinding, granite or slate quarrying or tunnelling. In the early stages small nodules are seen in the X-ray and such patients usually have no symptoms. Hilar nodes may contain a rim of ('eggshell') calcification. Silicosis is more likely than coal workers pneumoconiosis to increase even if there is no further exposure. Areas of massive fibrosis may develop, nodular shadowing may increase or upper lobe fibrosis may develop. At this stage effort dyspnoea is associated with the functional abnormalities of pulmonary fibrosis. There appears to be an increased risk of pulmonary tuberculosis.

Asbestos

Asbestos may have several different effects:

Diffuse pulmonary fibrosis – 'asbestosis'

Asbestosis (pulmonary fibrosis) occurs only after prolonged exposure to asbestos dusts. Symptoms of breathlessness on exertion may develop a few years after heavy exposure or many years after lighter exposure, (so that the patient may by then have forgotten that he once worked with asbestos-containing materials). Breathlessness, late inspiratory crackles on auscultation and often clubbing of the fingers resemble the features of fibrosing or extrinsic alveolitis (see Chapter 32) and lung function changes are also similar. Chest X-ray shows at first a bilateral 'ground glass' appearance in lower zones and later nodular shadows and loss of lung volume. Pleural changes of obliteration of costo-phrenic angles, or pleural plaques or calcification may be present and help distinguish asbestosis from other forms of diffuse fibrosis (see Chapter 32). Diagnosis rests on evidence of occupational exposure to asbestos, characteristic physical signs, X-ray appearances and lung function tests and on exclusion as far as possible of other causes of widespread fibrosis. The finding of asbestos bodies in sputum is merely evidence of exposure to asbestos and does not prove that an asbestos related-disease is present.

Pleural plaques (calcified or non-calcified)

Pleural plaques are seen on chest X-ray and cause no loss of function or symptoms. 45° oblique views may help to identify plaques.

Benign pleural effusion

Nearly always unilateral and recurrent, these occur in asbestos workers with or without other types of asbestos related disease. The fluid may be clear or blood stained and exclusion of other more sinister conditions such as lung cancer or pleural mesothelioma may be difficult.

Pleural fibrosis

Pleural fibrosis ('thickening') occurs in some asbestos workers, maybe as a sequel to repeated benign pleural effusions. If extensive, ventilation may be restricted and breathlessness result.

Malignant pleural (or peritoneal) mesothelioma

Malignant pleural mesothelioma (see p 181) may follow only light exposure which may not be occupational.

Carcinoma of the lung

Lung cancer is more common in patients with asbestosis (pulmonary fibrosis) than in the general population. The risk is increased many times further by cigarette smoking. It is not known whether asbestos workers who do not have asbestosis are at increased risk of lung cancer.

EXTRINSIC ALLERGIC ALVEOLITIS OF OCCUPATIONAL CAUSE (see also Chapter 32)

An occupational cause should always be considered. Suspicion is increased by:
1. work with a known cause of extrinsic allergic alveolitis (Table 36.3)
2. 'Clustering' of cases in one occupation or environment.

An occupational cause is more readily established for acute disease than in patients who are first seen with severe fibrosis, perhaps many years after a particular job.

Table 36.3 Some occupational causes of extrinsic allergic alveolitis

Condition	Source or organic dust
Farmer's lung	Mouldy hay
Mushroom worker's lung	Mushroom compost
Malt worker's lung	Mouldy barley
Bird fancier's lung	Droppings from pigeons, hens or other birds
'Ventilation pneumonia' or 'Humidifier fever'	Contaminated water in humidifiers

37 PULMONARY EOSINOPHILIA

Pulmonary eosinophilia is the association of abnormal pulmonary shadowing on chest X-ray with an excess of eosinophils in the peripheral blood. Eosinophilia may also occur without abnormalities on the chest X-ray particularly in patients with asthma.

Blood eosinophilia may occasionally accompany common conditions such as bronchial carcinoma, Hodgkins disease, sarcoidosis and tuberculosis. Its importance then is the risk that it may mislead, resulting in an incorrect diagnosis of one of the conditions more commonly associated with pulmonary eosinophilia.

AN APPROACH TO PULMONARY EOSINOPHILIA

If the patient has asthma

'Coincidental' eosinophilia
Many patients with asthma have a moderate blood eosinophilia which may persist if they develop unrelated lung conditions and may then cause diagnostic confusion.

Pulmonary eosinophilia in skin-test-positive asthma
Allergic bronchopulmonary aspergillosis (see page 171) is by far the commonest cause.

Pulmonary eosinophilia in skin-test-negative asthma
This is uncommon but should be considered when:
> — cough and breathlessness increase but, unlike the usual exacerbation of asthma, there is also malaise, fever and weight loss.
> — one or more features suggest additional non-respiratory disease, especially skin nodules, purpura, abdominal pain or arthralgia.

'Cryptogenic pulmonary eosinophilia'
May occur in asthmatics or non-asthmatics. Increased exertional breathlessness and non-productive cough are often associated with fever, sweating, weight loss and lassitude. This often leads to fruitless administration of antibiotics for presumed infection. Chest X-ray usually

shows either ill-defined patches of consolidation of non-segmental distribution especially in the upper zones or wide spread bilateral shadowing mainly in the upper zones. Eosinophilia may be slight or may exceed 10 000 per mm^3. ESR is raised and there is often a mild anaemia. Serum total IgE is not raised and tests for allergic aspergillosis (see page 171) are negative. There is a very rapid response of symptoms and X-ray to moderate doses of Prednisolone (20 mg daily).

Systemic vasculitis

This may occur in many clinical and pathological patterns and the classification and terminology are very confused. When pulmonary eosinophilia is associated with systemic vasculitis asthma has usually been present for some years often with perennial rhinitis, but may occur for the first time with onset of vasculitis.

Clues to diagnosis
>   — asthma may become more difficult to control
>   — increased effort breathlessness and dry cough may occur with
>   fever, weight-loss and debility
>   — abdominal pain or bloody diarrhoea
>   — purpura or skin nodules
>   — arthralgia or arthritis
>   — mononeuritis

Chest X-ray, though not abnormal in all patients with asthma and systemic vasculitis, in those with pulmonary eosinophilia may show either transient patchy 'pneumonic' shadows or widespread bilateral nodules. Blood eosinophil count is usually very high (over 8000 per mm^3) with high ESR and anaemia. Serum IgE levels are not raised.

Evidence of systemic vasculitis
>   — microscopic haematuria
>   — biopsy of skin lesions or of kidney
>   — possibly visceral angiography

In this setting biopsy of lung is not usually required but if evidence of pulmonary vasculitis is needed an open surgical biopsy is necessary to obtain a specimen of sufficient size to examine vessels.

Treatment with oral corticosteroids with or without cyclophosphamide may cause temporary improvement but the prognosis is usually poor especially if there is renal involvement.

If the patient does not have asthma

Consider

Parasitic infections

These usually, but not invariably, occur in those who have lived in areas of known high infestation. There may be few sysmptoms with slight cough, no wheeze and little or no fever. Unless eosinophilia or abnormal X-rays are noted the condition may pass unrecognized.

— examine stools for cysts and ova (ascaris, ankylostoma)
— serological tests are available for toxocara, toxoplasma, schistosomiasis and microfilaria (tropical eosinophilia). Levels of total IgE in blood are usually very high.

Drugs (see Chapter 35)

Cryptogenic pulmonary eosinophilia (see above)

Chronic eosinophilic pneumonia
An uncommon condition of unknown cause presenting with cough, fever, breathlessness and often weight loss which may persist for many weeks. It is not clear whether this is a different condition from cryptogenic pulmonary eosinophilia. Clues to the diagnosis are a typical X-ray appearance of consolidation involving predominantly the periphery of both lungs ('photographic negative of pulmonary oedema') and a high blood eosinophilia. If these characteristic features are present and tests for other causes of pulmonary eosinophilia are negative the diagnosis can be accepted without the need for lung biopsy. Treatment with oral steroids is usually rapidly effective but relapse may occur on reducing the dose.

38. THE ABNORMAL CHEST X-RAY

In this chapter an attempt is made to suggest an approach to diagnosis of patients who have some of the commoner radiographic abnormalities. In many patients the likely diagnosis will be apparent from the clinical history or physical examination or, conversely, these will exclude some of the possibilities which might be suggested on isolated examinations of the chest X-ray.

A chest X-ray may be found to be abnormal (a) while investigating the cause of respiratory symptoms, (b) while investigating non-respiratory symptoms, or (c) when, for some reason, an X-ray is taken of an apparently healthy person. Whilst sensible interpretation of abnormalities must take into account the reacons for which the films were taken, it is important to remember that the radiological abnormality may be unrelated to the respiratory or non-respiratory symptoms of which the patient complains.

SEGMENTAL OR LOBAR SHADOWING

This is shadowing occupying most or all of a lobe or segment (not merely a shadow within a particular lobe or segment). In order to recognise that a shadow or shadows are of lobar or segmental distribution it is essential that both PA and lateral views are examined. A knowledge of the anotomy of the bronchi and lobes and of the position of the fissures is also necessary. From knowledge of the space normally occupied by each lobe or segment it should be possible to decide whether there has been loss of volume associated with the abnormal shadowing.

Signs of loss of volume include:
— displacement of fissures
— displacement of mediastinum
— elevation of diaphragm
— displacement of hilar vessels
— crowding of ribs if volume loss is of large part of lung and is longstanding.

216

Volume of lobe or segment maintained

Acute illness
Pneumonia. In reality so called lobar pneumonia is rarely confined to one lobe and careful examination of the X-ray will often show shadowing transgressing lobar boundaries. An air bronchogram indicates consolidation and demonstrates that the airways to that portion of lung are patent.

Less acute illness
Consider infection beyond an obstructed or narrowed bronchus. If the bronchus is obstructed an air bronchogram will usually not be seen.

Loss of volume of a lobe or segment (collapse)

This suggests either obstruction of the bronchus or loss of lung volume during slow resolution of pneumonia (which may culminate in permanent loss of volume with fibrosis and bronchiectasis of the affected lobe or segment).

Diagnostic clues from the history

— Recent febrile illness suggests pneumonia
— Long-standing productive cough suggests bronchiectasis
— Haemoptysis suggests bronchial tumour or bronchiectasis
— Recent wheezing suggests localised bronchial narrowing.

Diagnostic clues from examination of the chest

— The 'classical' signs of consolidation are characteristic of (but infrequent in) acute bacterial pneumonia. More commonly fine inspiratory crackles are heard and, if there is a large area of consolidation, impairment of percussion note
— Coarse inspiratory crackles (with clubbing of fingers) suggests bronchiectasis
— Localised inspiratory or expiratory wheeze over radiologically abnormal lung suggests localised bronchial narrowing, as from a tumour or foreign body.

Further investigation

This will depend on the clinical setting.

Tomograms (see Chapter 6)
These may confirm that the shadowing is confined to a lobe or segment and may be used to show patency or obstruction of major bronchi. Segmental bronchi are usually less well shown on tomography. Tomography is no substitute for bronchoscopy if bronchial obstruction is suspected.

Bronchoscopy (see Chapter 10)
This allows direct examination of the bronchus proximal to a lobar or segmental abnormality, biopsy of any abnormality in the bronchus, aspiration of secretions and, if need be, biopsy of the abnormal lung tissue.

Bronchography (see Chapter 6)
This is required only if underlying bronchiectasis is suspected.

Persisting lobar or segmental shadowing with or without loss of volume and with or without an air bronchogram raises the possibility of bronchial obstruction and requires bronchoscopy.

SOLITARY LUNG MASS (Circumscribed opacity)

The problem

Malignant disease, primary or secondary, is the commonest cause in the middle aged and elderly whereas benign lesions are commoner than carcinoma in the young. Predicting either of these with certainty is very difficult or impossible. The problem therefore is whether to recommend surgical removal, biopsy of the lesion or observation by repeated X-rays.

Symptoms

The most difficult problems of diagnosis and management are in patients who have no symptoms. Lung masses themselves rarely cause local symptoms unless they are large enough to destroy or displace much of the lung or they compress or invade adjacent structures.

— An acute or sub-acute febrile illness suggests abscess
— Haemoptysis suggests primary malignancy
— Weight loss suggests malignancy or abscess.

History

— Has the patient had a previous chest X-ray? Was it abnormal? Can it be obtained? (It is not uncommon for a small opacity to be recognised on a previous X-ray having been originally overlooked)
— Is, or was, the patient a cigarette smoker? Primary bronchial carcinoma is uncommon in non-smokers
— Any known previous tumours (including uterine fibroids or 'benign' tumours of skin or elsewhere)?
— Any symptoms of rheumatoid arthritis? Rheumatoid nodules may be single or multiple.

Clinical examination

This usually yields few clues.

- Examine carefully for enlargement of lymph nodes and examine other common sites of metastases (liver, skin)
- Carefully palpate breasts, thyroid, prostate, testes and ovaries for a small, previous unnoticed primary tumour
- Clubbing of the fingers suggests malignancy or abscess.

The chest X-ray

- Are any previous films available? Was the lesion present and, if so, has it changed?
- Is the lesion genuine and in the lung (e.g. not a nipple or a skin papilloma)?
- Is the lesion calcified? Central or laminar calcification indicates a benign lesion. Calcification may be apparent on the plain radiograph but is better demonstrated by tomography
- Is the lesion truly solitary? Conventional tomography of the whole of both lungs or, better, computed tomography may demonstrate other shadows (suggesting metastases)
- Has it changed in size? If previous films are available and the opacity has not enlarged over 2 years malignancy is unlikely (but by no means impossible)
- What is the shape and outline of the opacity? An irregular or lobulated outline suggests primary carcinoma, and sharp outline favours either a benign tumour or a metastasis but these are not reliable signs. Characterstic feeding or draining vessels suggest a vascular malformation.

Other investigations

- A radiological search for a primary tumour (barium studies, IVU etc) is expensive, time-consuming and usually fruitless but it is easy to examine urine for microscopic haematuria (renal carcinoma)
- Peripheral blood count and ESR rarely contribute to diagnosis
- Other blood investigations (rheumatoid factor, complement-fixation tests for fungal or hydatid disease) are performed if indicated by history or clinical examination.

Management

If, as is usually the case, there are no reliable indications that the lesion is benign, a decision must be made whether to remove the lesion surgically, attempt biopsy or observe with serial X-rays.

— If the patient is under the age of 40 a benign lesion is most likely; biopsy may be performed (percutaneous needle biopsy or transbronchial biopsy depending on the size and site of opacity and the locally available expertise) or the lesion may be observed on serial X-rays

— If the patient is over the age of 40 malignancy is more likely. Biopsy is justified only if the result will influence subsequent management (that is it will avoid the need for thoracotomy). In centres with experienced personnel biopsy of solitary lesions yields useful information in 80–90% of patients but is more reliable for confirming carcinoma than for establishing the exact nature of a benign lesion. On occasions however characteristic features of a benign lesion, such as a hamartoma, or demonstration of tubercle bacilli in biopsy material, may allow a firm diagnosis to be made.

UNILATERAL RAISED DIAPHRAGM

— Is the degree of elevation abnormal and consistent? It is wise to repeat the X-ray, ensuring that the patient has taken a full inspiration, before concluding that an abnormality is present

— Is it really a raised diaphragm? Consider the possibility that the appearances are due to a subpulmonary pleural effusion (decubitus or supine film will usually help), collapse or consolidation of the middle and lower lobe, a large pleural or intrapulmonary mass in the lower chest, or a mass beneath the diaphragm

— Are previous films available? Is this a recent or long standing abnormality?

If it is a raised diaphragm

— Is it an isolated abnormality?
— Is there any pleural fluid?
— Is there any evidence of lobar collapse on that side? (to account for the raised diaphragm)
— Is there a hilar mass?
— Is the diaphragm paralysed? This is most easily decided by 'screening' by fluoroscopy and observing movements of the two diaphragms during deep inspiration or on sniffing.

If diaphragm is paralysed

— Are there any radiographic clues to the cause? Bronchial carcinoma is the most common and, in this situation a mass

can usually be seen on careful examination of PA and lateral chest films. If in doubt conventional or computerised tomography are rarely helpful
— Is there any history or sign of recent herpes zoster of C4 distribution?
— Is there any history of trauma to the neck or any evidence of neurological (bronchial plexus or cervical cord) disease?

If the diaphragm is not paralysed

Is there any history or sign to suggest abdominal conditions, (liver abscess or tumour, subphrenic collection, renal tumours, ascites or late pregnancy) which may either push the diaphragm up or inhibit its movement?

It may be difficult or impossible to identify the cause of an isolated elevated diaphragm. Bronchoscopy very seldom reveals a cause if the chest X-ray is otherwise normal and thoracotomy is difficult to justify as malignant disease involving the phrenic nerve would be incurable by operation.

PLEURAL OPACITIES

Pleural fluid

Recognition is not difficult in most patients as the radiographic appearances are characteristic. Sub-pulmonary effusion may however simulate an elevated diaphragm. Effusions encysted within the fissures may mimic an intrapulmonary mass but the shape and position of the shadow on PA and lateral views should arouse suspicion of pleural fluid and there is usually but not always a small quantity of free pleural fluid visible on such X-rays.

Pleural 'thickening'

This term is often used imprecisely to imply fibrosis of the pleura. Uncritical acceptance of this diagnosis may lead to overlooking an effusion, pleural tumour or empyema. Fibrotic thickening of the pleura can usually be differentiated from fluid on decubitus films but localised collections of fluid adjacent to the chest wall may be difficult to distinguish from solid pleural masses on plain X-rays. Ultrasound or computed tomography may then be required for diagnosis.

Pleural masses

Benign pleural tumours are uncommon and malignant tumours usually cause a pleural effusion. It is important to consider the possibility of empyema if a pleural mass is seen in a patient who is unwell, losing weight or has had a recent respiratory infection. A haematoma or callus around a rib fracture may simulate a pleural mass. Benign pleural plaques, usually but not always related to asbestos exposure, are almost invariably multiple and bilateral.

Pleural calcification

Extensive pleural calcification may follow a haemothorax or long-standing tuberculous empyema. Localised, and often multiple, areas of calcification (including linear calcification of the diaphragmatic pleura) may follow asbestos exposure.

Further investigations of pleural opacities

Aspiration or biopsy
For investigation of pleural fluid see Chapter 27. If the lesion appears to be solid, biopsy by any of the percutaneous techniques described in Chapter 11 or by limited thoracotomy may be necessary.

DIFFUSE LUNG SHADOWING

We suggest here an approach to the problem of a patient in whom widespread lung shadowing is the main or an outstanding feature. We will not attempt to offer a comprehensive list of causes but will confine ourselves the the commoner conditions encountered in the UK.

Radiographic features including the size, shape, density and distribution of opacities may in themselves suggest the more likely diagnoses and we strongly recommend consultation with a radiologist who is aware of the patient's symptoms before embarking on investigations other than the most straightforward.

In general such patients fall into one or three categories:
— No respiratory symptoms (chest radiograph was taken for some other reason)
— Recent onset of symptoms (usually breathlessness)
— Long-standing symptoms (usually breathlessness).
Although these subdivisions are clearly artificial they provide useful guidance to the conditions which must be considered and hence a sensible approach to investigation.

No respiratory symptoms

The duration of the radiological abnormality can rarely be established unless chest X-rays have, for some reason, been taken in the past. The commonest causes are sarcoidosis (see Chapter 33) or pneumoconiosis (see Chapter 36). The presence of bilateral hilar lymph node enlargement or right paratracheal node enlargement greatly increases the probability of sarcoidosis but lymph nodes are frequently not enlarged when widespread shadowing is present. There are usually no abnormal findings on clinical examination of the lungs.

Pneumoconioses from non-fibrogenic mineral dusts (such as coal or silica) usually produce no abnormal respiratory signs, and no clubbing. Pneumoconioses from fibrogenic dusts (such as asbestos) may produce inspiratory crackles and clubbing of fingers.

Recent onset of symptoms

Infection
In a patient with normal host defences it is very unusual for primary bacterial pneumonia to produce bilateral diffuse widespread shadowing and patients thus affected would be extremely ill and very breathless. An important exception is miliary tuberculosis in which numerous very small nodules of similar size are scattered throughout both lung fields in a patient who may not, at least initially, appear to be very ill and who may not be breathless. Pneumonia complicating measles or chicken pox may produce widespread nodular shadows and a similar appearance sometimes occurs in infection with *mycoplasma pneumoniae* or *legionella* or with opportunist infections (see Chapter 20).

Alveolitis
In cryptogenic fibrosing alveolitis (see Chapter 32) fine late inspiratory crackles can be heard but clubbing may not yet have developed. Such patients are usually breathless on exertion.

In extrinsic allergic alveolitis (see Chapter 32) the history of exposure is all-important. Fine late inspiratory crackles are usually, but not invariably, heard. Fever, malaise and weight loss, together with a neutrophil leucocytosis, may erroneously suggest infection.

Left ventricular failure
Evidence of primary heart disease is usually apparent and the heart is usually seen to be enlarged on the X-ray.

Alveolar haemorrhage
This (as in Goodpasture's syndrome) is usually but not always accompanied by haemoptysis.

Malignancy
Haematogenous metastases may be seen as numerous small nodules, and lymphangitis carcinomatosa produces septal lines, sometimes with enlarged mediastinal nodes. There may also be pleural effusions.

Drug induced lung disease (see Chapter 35)
This history will reveal treatment with cytotoxic or other drugs which are known to produce widespread lung changes; peripheral blood eosinophilia will be a clue to pulmonary eosinophilic responses to drugs.

Pulmonary eosinophilia (see Chapter 37)

Long-standing symptoms

Fibrogenic mineral dust inhalation (e.g. asbestos)
An occupational history, inspiratory crackles and clubbing of fingers may be present and there may be associated pleural plaques or calcification (see Chapter 36).

Fibrosing alveolitis
See Chapter 32 and above.

Bronchiectasis
There is usually a history of long-standing cough with purulent sputum and perhaps haemoptysis. Often 'ring shadows' are seen on X-ray.

Chronic aspiration pneumonia
There is often, but not always, a history of swallowing difficulties with a demonstrable cause (achalasia, bulbar weakness etc).

Further investigations

A blood count may show leucocytosis in bacterial infection or extrinsic allergic alveolitis, eosinophilia in drug reactions or pulmonary eosinophilia, and a very high ESR may suggest a connective tissue disorder. If tuberculosis or malignancy seem likely sputum (if obtainable) should be examined for tubercle bacilli and malignant cells. Circulating precipitins against avian proteins or the antigens of farmers lung should be sought if the history suggests extrinsic allergic alveolitis of such a cause. Anti-nuclear factor or rheumatoid factor may be found in the blood in cryptogenic fibrosing alveolitis, asbestosis or systemic lupus erythematosis. If sarcoidosis is suspected and there is no urgency for diagnosis the Kviem test may be of value (see Chapter 33).

Having considered these and rarer possibilities the diagnosis may be fairly certain so that treatment, if required, may be started. More often, one is left with a 'short list' of probable causes and a decision must be made about the need for histological and perhaps microbiological examination of the lung by lung biopsy. The decision whether or not to biopsy and, if so, which technique to choose, is often difficult.
— Can the diagnosis be made with confidence without biopsy?
— Is biopsy likely to confirm (or exclude) a condition requiring specific therapy such as miliary tuberculosis, disseminated malignancy, pneumocystis infection, alveolar proteinosis or sarcoidosis, or to help in giving a prognosis?
— If one of the many fibrotic or fibrosing processes seems certain, will the findings on lung biopsy distinguish between them, guide therapy or prognosis, or influence management or outcome? This question is often difficult to answer as most such patients will receive a trial of treatment with oral cortocosteroids and it could be argued that the outcome depends more on the response to this treatment than on the histological appearances.

The choice of method of biopsy is discussed in Chapter 11 and is a matter for decision by those experienced in the management of this type of chest disease and in biopsy procedures.

MEDIASTINAL MASSES

The site of the radiological abnormality will immediately suggest possible origins of the mass (Fig. 38.1). In the absence of symptoms which suggest more direct methods of investigation (e.g. stridor, dysphagia) the first exercise is to determine radiographically the site and characteristics of the mass. This process has been greatly simplified by computed tomography but conventional tomography, barium swallow or aortography may be useful in the absence of computed tomography. If aortic aneurysm and achalasia of the oesophagus have been excluded most isolated masses, whether in the anterior, middle or posterior mediastinum, which on radiographic appearance are unlikely to represent enlarged lymph nodes, will require surgical removal.

Intrathoracic lymph node enlargement

Bilateral symmetrical enlargement of hilar nodes, especially if associated with paratracheal node enlargement in an asymptomatic young adult, strongly suggests sarcoidosis. Investigations to confirm the diagnosis are

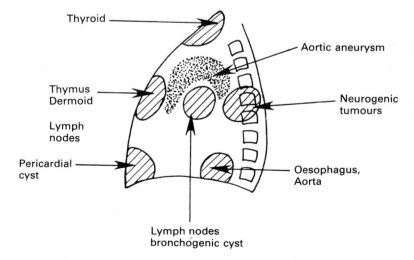

Fig. 38.1 Some mediastinal opacities on a lateral chest X-ray

discussed in Chapter 33. Similar appearances in a patient who is ill may be due to lymphoma but the enlargement of nodes is usually asymmetrical.

Unilateral hilar node enlargement is rarely due to sarcoidosis. More common causes are Hodgkin's disease, lymph node metastasese from an inapparent bronchial carcinoma or tumour of the genitourinary tract or, in those of Asian origin or in children, tuberculosis.

Having searched for enlarged lymph nodes elsewhere or other evidence of disseminated disease, histological examination of tissue may be necessary for diagnosis. In sarcoidosis this can often be obtained from bronchoscopic biopsy of bronchial mucosa or transbronchial biopsy of lung tissue (see Chapter 11). Tuberculosis may be strongly suspected from the association of intrathoracic lymph nodes and a strongly positive tuberculin test in an Asian but additional proof of the diagnosis may be considered necessary before starting treatment. Mediastinoscopy is of most value when the radiologically enlarged nodes are seen in the upper or mid mediastinum, but the diagnosis may be obtained from biopsy of nodes which are not sufficiently enlarged to be visible on chest X-ray or tomography (but such nodes are often seen to be enlarged on CT). Hilar nodes may be biopsied by the relatively minor surgical procedure of anterior mediastinotomy. Formal thoracotomy may be required to remove or biopsy other lymph node or tumour masses.

Section 4
SOME ASPECTS OF
TREATMENT

39. OXYGEN THERAPY

Uses

Oxygen enrichment of inspired air has the sole purpose of correcting hypoxia. Oxygen is of no therapeutic value in the absence of hypoxia. (The only exception is the use of oxygen as a convenient method of nebulising drugs.)

Principles

Room air at sea level contains 21% oxygen. Increasing the proportion of oxygen raises the tension of oxygen in alveoli and thereby increases arterial oxygen tension (Pa_{O2}). The rise of Pa_{O2} is less than would occur in a healthy subject if there is mismatching of ventilation and perfusion in the lungs as is often the case in patients who require oxygen therapy. Only a small increase of Pa_{O2} can be achieved from oxygen therapy in the presence of a large right to left shunt (as for example in some forms of congenital heart disease) or in conditions such as pneumonia in which large portions of lung are perfused but not ventilated.

Clinical indications

The main clinical uses of oxygen are discussed in Chapter 39.

Note: Oxygen is a useful but potentially dangerous drug and should be prescribed with the same thought and consideration of dosage as any other powerful drug. It is not a harmless 'tonic' to be given at the whim of untrained staff.

SUPPLY OF OXYGEN

Piped oxygen is available in most hospital wards with flow meters which permit flows of up to 10 l/min. Standard cylinders contain either 1360 or 3400 litres of compressed oxygen. Small portable cylinders containing 240 l of oxygen can be filled through a special valve from a larger cylinder. Liquid oxygen systems are under trial for portable oxygen therapy. Oxygen concentrators which separate oxygen from the other constituents of air offer the least expensive method of providing continuous oxygen in the home. They can however deliver no more than about 4 l/min.

Flow regulators

The flow regulatory device on standard wall fittings and cylinders permit delivery in the range 0–10 l/min. Most portable oxygen cylinders and the cylinders supplied for home use in UK are fitted with a fixed-flow regulator which delivers 2 l/min on the 'medium' setting and 4 l/min on 'high' setting. The term 'low' is presumably avoided on psychological grounds. It is important to note that these low flows are insufficient to drive most commercially available nebulisers (see Chapter 41) and for some of the venturi-type masks.

Oxygen delivery

This is achieved through a mask or nasal cannulae. Oxygen tents are rarely used in adult practice.

Masks

Masks cover the nose and mouth and earlier versions carried the risk of causing rebreathing of exhaled carbon dioxide.

The MC mask

This consists of a transparent plastic cone with oxygen fed into its apex. Holes around the inflow pipe allow for inhalation of room air and for expiration. With 1 litre of oxygen the concentration in the mask is about 28% and at a flow of 6 litres of oxygen the mask concentration reaches about 60%. As with all attempts to deliver high concentrations of oxygen, the MC mask becomes less reliable when the very high inspiratory flows of a very breathless patient exceed the output from the mask so that such patients inhale considerably lower concentrations of oxygen than those measured under usual conditions. The dead space of the MC mask, although not large, results in a tendency to rebreathe CO_2 which is undesirable in treatment of patients with hypercapnia.

The Edinburgh mask

This consists of a loose plastic face piece into which an oxygen pipe projects laterally. At a flow of 1 l/min it gives a mask concentration of 25–29%; a concentration of 31–35% at 2 l/min and 33–39% at 3 l/min. CO_2 retention does not seem to occur.

Venturi masks

These (e.g. the 'Ventimask') consist of a light plastic cone at the apex of which is a small jet through which oxygen enters, air being entrained through adjacent ports by the Venturi principle. The concentration of oxygen in the mask depends on the size of the ports and to only a slight extent on the flow of oxygen.

Standard masks produce oxygen concentrations of 24%, 28%, 35%, 40% and 60%. The minimum oxygen inflow recommended by manufacturers to yield these concentrations and produce sufficient total volume of oxygen-enriched air are 2, 4, 8, 10 and 15 litres per minute respectively. If the patient is hyperventilating higher oxygen flows are recommended to increase the total output (but these flows often cannot be delivered using the standard flow meters in many wards and on cylinders, which deliver a maximum of 10 l/min). Even at the highest normally attainable oxygen inflow the hyperventilating patient will dilute the mask output with room air and will therefore receive a mouth oxygen concentration below that stated on the 60% Venturi mask. At lower concentrations however these masks are reliable and accurate and they are comfortable to wear.

Nasal cannulae

These 'prongs' deliver oxygen directly into the nose through twin plastic cannulae placed in the anterior nares. The inspired oxygen concentration cannot be set or measured precisely. At a flow of 1 l/min they produce changes in arterial oxygen tension equivalent to inhalation of 25–30% oxygen, at 2 l/min equivalent to 30–35% and at 3 l/min equivalent to 32–38%. The concentration received by the patient varies somewhat with mouth or nose breathing, or with nasal obstruction. Nasal cannulae are not successful for delivering high concentrations of oxygen, even at high oxygen flows.

Nasal cannulae are comfortable and have the unique advantage that oxygen can be delivered continuously without the need to interrupt treatment as occurs when a patient wearing a mask wishes to expectorate, eat, drink or wash.

Humidification

Prolonged inhalation of dry gas can disturb ciliary action and cause dryness or crusting of the mouth or nose in addition to causing fluid loss as dry gas is humidified in the respiratory tract. These effects are important however, only if the upper respiratory tract is bypassed as when a patient has an endotracheal tube or tracheostomy.

Humidification is not required if oxygen is delivered by mask at low concentrations. If high flows are delivered for a long period by nasal cannulae or possibly by mask, humidification may reduce discomfort but is not easy to achieve. Heated humidifiers are more effective than bubbling oxygen through cold water but carry the risk of bacterial contamination, and much of the water taken up tends to condense in the tubing before reaching the patient.

RISKS AND TOXICITY OF OXYGEN THERAPY

— The risks of uncontrolled oxygen therapy in treatment of chronic or acute hypercapneic respiratory failure are discussed in Chapter 16
— Fortunately none of the available delivery systems offers 100% oxygen to the spontaneously breathing patient, and concentrations above 60% are attained only during assisted ventilation. At concentrations above 60% pulmonary oxygen toxicity may cause pulmonary oedema or areas of subsegmental collapse
— It has been suggested that pulmonary toxicity of certain drugs such as bleomycin (see Chapter 35) is increased by administration of oxygen
— Oxygen is combustible. Patients receiving oxygen must not smoke or light matches, a point of special importance when oxygen is provided in the home.

SOME SPECIAL USES OF OXYGEN

Long-term domiciliary oxygen therapy (see also Chapter 29)

This has been shown in several studies to prolong life of certain patients with chronic hypoxia due to chronic bronchitis and emphysema. The more hours in the day that oxygen is taken the better the survival figures but it seems that a minimum of 15 hours in every 24 is necessary for any beneficial effect. Oxygen is taken throughout the night to counter the fall of Pa_{O_2} which occurs in such patients during sleep. Fifteen hours of treatment also entails using oxygen for some of the waking hours, but some patients continue at daytime work throughout this treatment.

At present long-term oxygen therapy should be considered for some patients with chronic bronchitis and emphysema with severe airflow obstruction and:
— hypoxia (Pa_{O_2} below 7 kPa) on several occasions measured during the day with the patient in a steady state
— evidence of complications of hypoxia such as peripheral oedema, right ventricular hypertrophy or ECG on or secondary polycythaemia
— there is no rise of Pa_{CO_2} during administration of oxygen at sufficient concentration to raise Pa_{O_2} above 10 KPa.

Some would also insist that the patient no longer smoked both because of the risk of fire in the home and also because of the possibility that smoking may reduce the benefits of the treatment.

Oxygen is most conveniently and most cheaply provided by an oxygen concentrator at a rate of 1–3 l/min by nasal prongs, to achieve a Pa_{O_2} greater than 10 KPa. Failing this at least fourteen 1344 litre oxygen cylinders must be delivered to the patient's home each week. Liquid oxygen systems are also being developed.

Oxygen must be piped to the patient's bed and, in order to achieve 15 hours a day, to one or more living rooms in the house. The practical difficulties are self-evident and it is likely that this form of treatment, even if effective, will be practicable for only a very small proportion of all patients who fultil the criteria suggested.

Portable oxygen

Portable oxygen may reduce the breathlessness and increase the exercise capacity of some patients with chronic lung disease. It has been most widely used for patients with chronic bronchitis but may benefit breathless patients with pulmonary fibrosis or small or stiff lungs of other cause. It is, of course, essential that all other aspects of treatment such as optimal bronchodilator therapy are also given.

It is not possible to predict which patients will benefit and we recommend measuring exercise capacity (see Chapter 7), with an assessment by the patient of perceived breathlessness during exercise with and without additional oxygen (1–2 l/min). The element of suggestion is so great that the patient should receive either air or additional oxygen by nasal cannulae during both periods of exercise and neither the patient nor the investigator should know which gas is being given during each test.

Only if clear benefit is apparent are the costs and inconveniences of portable oxygen justified. It must be remembered that some of the benefits of supplement oxygen during exercise are countered by the weight of a portable cylinder. Patients receiving long-term oxygen may enjoy freedom to leave their home if supplied with portable oxygen.

40. NEBULISATION OF DRUGS

Definition
Nebulisation is the formation of an aerosol by the passage of a gas through a liquid.

Nebulizing systems

There are two methods of nebulisation:

Ultrasonic
These are expensive and produce the same range of particle size as jet nebulisers but have a higher output which may cause fluid overload. These machines have no advantages over the jet nebulisers.

Jet nebulisers
In this type of nebuliser gas is expelled through a fine nozzle above a capillary tube which has its base in the liquid to be nebulised. By the Bernouilli effect pressure falls where the velocity of gas increases at its exit from the nozzle, and liquid is drawn up the capillary tube into this area of low pressure. The liquid is blown by the jet of air against a baffle which breaks particles into a smaller size. Any liquid particles which are not converted into an aerosol drop back into the reservoir of liquid at the bottom of the nebuliser and in time are sucked up the capillary tube again. Those particles which remain as an aerosol can be inspired by the patient.

The ideal particle size for therapeutic nebulisation is 1 to 10 microns but particles may change size within the airways due to their electrical charge, hygroscopic effects due to the humidity of the gas in the airways and coalescence of the particles. It has been customary to use about 2 ml solution in order to limit the duration of treatment to about 10 minutes but dilution to 4 ml lessens aerosol deposition on the walls of the nebuliser resulting in a larger dose reaching the patient.

Either a face mask or mouth piece may be used to deliver the aerosol to the patient. A face mask is often easier for ill patients but a slightly higher dose is delivered through the mouth piece, which may also be more convenient for children.

Various sources of compressed gas are available. In the past oxygen cylinders have frequently been used but these are often not satisfactory because:

234

— high concentrations of oxygen may be dangerous to patients with chronic lung disease (see Chapter 16)

— domiciliary oxygen cylinders generate a flow rate of only 2–4 litres and most nebulisers require a flow of at least 6–8 litres/minute to produce a sufficient output of correctly sized particles.

The best source of gas is an air compressor. These are usually electrically powered pumps, but foot pumps and hand nebulisers are also available.

Many different designs of nebulisers and compressors are available commercially. It is important to ensure that the compressor delivers sufficient airflow for the nebuliser chosen.

Intermittent positive pressure nebulisation has been widely used in the past but the equipment is expensive, the controls are complicated and the positive pressure may force air in to damaged parts of the lungs, hence increasing ventilation-perfusion imbalance. Positive pressure nebulisation does not give better deliver of aerosol than a compressor which delivers aerosol at atmospheric pressure. Administration of nebulised drugs by positive pressure equipment is advantageous only if the patient is so weak or tired that positive pressure usefully reduces the work of inspiration.

Nebulisable drugs

A variety of drugs may be nebulised. These fall into the following main groups.

Bronchodilators
Bronchodilators and cromoglycate are frequently nebulised for the prevention or treatment of asthma (see Chapter 30).

Antibiotics
These may sterilise expectorated secretions but probably have little effect on treating either bronchial infection or pneumonia. They may be of some benefit in cystic fibrosis (see Chapter 23). Nebulised amphotericin has been used in treatment of aspergillomas but the drug is not effective unless administered directly into the mycetoma cavity.

'Mucolytics'
These have been used extensively in the past. They may reduce the viscosity and elasticity of sputum but rarely seem to improve either symptoms or lung function.

Local anaesthetics
Local anaesthetics (e.g. lignocaine), may occasionally be given to suppress a troublesome cough for which no serious underlying cause has been found.

41. INSERTION OF AN INTERCOSTAL TUBE

Indications for intercostal tubes

Pneumothorax
See Chapter 26 for indications.

Pleural effusion
Small pleural effusions can be completely aspirated without the need to leave an intercostal tube in place but larger effusions usually need either intermittent or continuous drainage through an indwelling tube (see Chapter 27). The intercostal tube can also be used for irrigation in treatment of empyemas (see Chapter 27).

Sites of insertion of intercostal drain

Pneumothorax
The preferred site of insertion of the drain is in the mid-axillary line in about the 3rd intercostal space which is on the same horizontal level as the 4th costo-chondral joint anteriorly. If this site is not suitable because of tethering of the pleura to the chest wall, the tube can be inserted anteriorly in the 2nd intercostal space in the mid clavicular line (lateral to the internal mammary artery).

Pleural effusion
It is much more common for an intercostal drain to be inserted too low than too high, with the risk of perforating the liver, spleen or stomach. Pleural fluid is present well above the level of dullness on percussion and above the apparent upper level of fluid on the PA chest X-ray. Only in exceptional circumstances should an intercostal drain be inserted below the inferior angle of the scapula. A site near the top of the area of dullness is usually best. If the effusion is loculated careful calculation of the site of the fluid from chest X-ray, ultrasound or CT examination may help in selecting the correct site for insertion of the drain.

Technique of insertion of intercostal drain

1. Select correct tube size. Large bore tubes are advisable if the effusion is likely to be bloody or an empyema and if the drain is to be left in site for a prolonged period. Narrower

236

drains are satisfactory for transudates and pneumothoraces. The range of intercostal drains is 16–32 gauge and the transparent, plastic tubes (e.g. Argyll or Portex) are satisfactory

2. Explain the procedure to the patient and reassure him. Assess the need for sedation (e.g. intravenous diazepam)
3. Select the site for insertion of the drain and mark it in ink
4. Position the patient so that he is comfortable and you have good access to the site of insertion of the drain. The patient should be sitting forwards resting on pillows on a support
5. Sterilise the skin surrounding the insertion site with antiseptic (e.g. iodine)
6. Inject 1 or 2% lignocaine as local anaesthetic subcutaneously and then deeper through the chest wall. The anaesthetic should be given right down to the pleura and at this level intermittent aspiration will confirm when the needle has penetrated into the pleural cavity. It is safe to insert the tube to drain fluid or air only if fluid or air respectively are obtained at this stage
7. With a scalpel initially, then with artery forceps, dissect the tissues down to the pleura so that a track which is the size of the tube to be inserted is made right through the tissues of the chest wall
8. Insert the trocar down this track and with a twisting motion *gently* push it through the pleura. *It should not be necessary to push hard on the trocar if blunt dissection has been adequate beforehand.* If the intercostal space appears smaller than the tube it is helpful to ask the patient to take a deep inspiration and even to flex their spine away from the operator to enlarge the intercostal space. When the resistance of the pleura has been overcome push the tube apically if a pneumothorax is to be drained or basally if a pleural effusion is to be drained
9. Connect the tube to an underwater seal for a pneumothorax (see Chapter 26) or to a closed-circuit collecting system for a pleural effusion. With a pneumothorax air should be seen to bubble through the underwater seal and with a pleural effusion the fluid should be visible down the conducting tube. An underwater seal acts as a one-way valve which allows air out of the chest but not in. It is of course essential that the end of the tube from the chest is under the surface of the water, but the tip should be less than 2 cm below the surface lest the hydrostatic pressure of the column of water resists escape of air from the tube. The level of water in the bottle should be measured so that the volume of fluid draining through the intercostal tube can be calculated

10. Insert one or two stitches to close the wound if necessary and another stitch across the middle of the wound which is left untied. This will be used to close the opening when the tube is removed. Fix yet another stitch in the skin and tie its free ends tightly and repeatedly round the tube to anchor it in position. Remember that the fixation stitich is likely to cut through the skin within about a week. If the tube is left for longer than this it must be fixed by adhesive strapping. For this purpose take a length of narrow strapping 50 cm long and wrap its mid-portion around the tube several times at the point where the tube emerges from the skin. Fix the ends to the chest wall so that they lie in a straight line. Take another similar length of strapping, fix it to the tube and then to the chest wall at right angles to the first strip

11. Arrange a chest X-ray to check the position of the tube.

Removal of intecostal drain

This requires two people. The patient is asked to breathe in and then slowly breathe out. One person removes the tube quickly and applies an occlusive dressing while the other ties the suture to prevent air entering the pleural cavity. The occlusive dressing can be removed after 48 hours.

Use of suction (see also Chapter 26)

Suction may be required for pneumothoraces which fail to expand with intercostal intubation alone. In the presence of a functioning drain, failure of a pneumothorax to improve indicates that more air is leaking into the pleural cavity than is being removed through the drain. This can often be overcome by increasing air flow through the tube by applying a negative pressure to the distal end. This is achieved by a low pressure high volume pump and, if this fails, by insertion of a second tube, which can be connected by a Y connector to the underwater seal. The pressure gauges on suction are marked in various units but suction of 25–50 cm of water is usually sufficient.

The importance of using a pump which can deal with high volumes of air cannot be over-emphasised. Low volume pumps producing a high vacuum are useless in treating a pneumothorax and may even be dangerous by limiting the volume of air which can escape from the chest.

42. ENDOTRACHEAL INTUBATION

Endotracheal intubation is a practical skill. Staff who may need to intubate patients should contact their anaesthetist colleagues to arrange for practical instruction.

Indications

— Severe upper airways obstruction e.g. acute epiglottitis (in treating this group of patients it is desirable to have a skilled anaesthetist and facilities for tracheostomy immediately available)
— Protection of the tracheo-bronchial tree in patients in coma or where the competence of the larynx is impaired
— To facilitate intermittent positive pressure ventilation, during anaesthesia, following cardiac arrest, in the treatment of drug overdosage and in the general management of patients with hypoventilation or gross ventilation perfusion mismatch
— Access to the tracheo-bronchial tree for aspiration of secretions. This is rarely the sole indication for intubation. Bronchoscopy can be used for 'acute' aspiration and crico-thyroid cannulation (mini-tracheostomy) for 'chronic' indications
— Specific anaesthetic indications e.g. to allow surgery on the head and neck or operations in the prone position.

Equipment

1. Laryngoscope, preferably Mackintosh pattern. Check batteries and bulb
2. Endotracheal tube of suitable size. (9.0 mm for adult male, 8.0 mm for adult female, range of tubes for paediatric cases. Rough guide for paediatric tube: size in mm = age/4 + 4.5)
   Connector for endotracheal tube
   Catheter mount to connect to resuscitation bag
   Syringe and clamp for inflatable cuff
   Introducer with flexible tip
   Syringe for inflating cuff

Lubricating gel
Tape to secure tube
3. Suction apparatus with pharyngeal sucker and appropriate
   endotracheal suction catheters. *Note*: external diameter of
   suction catheter should not be greater than half the internal
   diameter of the endotracheal tube (e.g. 12 FG for 8 and
   9 mm tubes)
4. Resuscitation bag (Leardal or Ambu), suitable masks and
   airways
5. If the patient's level of consciousness will not permit
   intubation suitable drugs to produce hypnosis (e.g.
   thiopentone, methohexitone, diazepam) and muscular
   relaxation (e.g. suxamethonium, alcuronium) will be needed.

Technique

1. Position the head with the neck flexed and the head
   extended, ('sniffing the morning air')
2. Hold the laryngoscope in the left hand and introduce the
   blade into the right side of the mouth taking care to avoid
   damaging the lips. Advance the blade, sweeping the tongue
   to the left. When using the laryngoscope there should be no
   pressure on the teeth; the lifting action to visualise the larynx
   should be applied at right angles to the blade in the direction
   of the axis of the handle. When the uvula has been identified
   lift up the handle of the laryngoscope while advancing the
   blade. Identify the epiglottis at this stage and advance the
   blade anterior to the epiglottis while continuing to lift the
   handle. The larynx should now be visible and the
   endotracheal tube can be passed between the cords.
      If the larynx is not seen:
   a. Has the laryngoscope been passed into the oesophagus?
      Withdraw slightly and identify the epiglottis
   b. Ask an assistant to press the larynx backwards to bring it
      into view
   c. Pass an introducer through the tube. With two or three
      inches of introducer sticking out of the distal end of the
      tube gentle attempts can be made to find the larynx. Once
      the introducer is in the larynx the tube can be advanced
      over the introducer
3. Confirm that the endotracheal tube is in the trachea.
   a. Press on the chest whilst listening over the end of the tube
      to detect air movement
   b. Connect the resuscitation bag and confirm that the chest
      expands when the bag is compressed
   c. Check breath sounds over both lungs while compressing
      the resuscitation bag

4. The cuff on the tube should be inflated with just enough air to prevent an air leak during inflation. Over-inflation can lead to necrosis of the tracheal wall. Check breath sounds over both lungs after inflating the cuff. If they are unequal adjust the position of the tube which is probably too far in
5. Fix the tube to prevent displacement
6. Leave the tube connected to the resuscitation bag or connect to a ventilator or other circuit as appropriate
7. If longer term intubation intended check the position of the tube with a chest X-ray.

Problems with intubation

Common causes of difficulty with oral intubation are:
Doctor — inexperience
Patient — short neck
— cervical spine disease
— receding chin
— protruding teeth
— gross obesity
— inflammation and oedema in pharynx

Complications

Trauma
— Broken teeth. Lift the laryngoscope handle – don't use the blade as a lever on the teeth
— Trauma to lips, tongue, pharynx or larynx. Avoid by taking reasonable care
— Tracheal trauma. Inflate the cuff carefully, check for correct volume of air.

No lung ventilation
— Intubation of right main bronchus. Suspect if inflation pressure rises; check air entry over left lung. Adjust position of tube
— Obstruction. Check for kinking of tube. Check tube not obstructed with secretions by passing suction catheter. If obstruction cannot be overcome extubate and either reintubate or ventilate patient with mask, airway and resuscitation bag.

Management of the intubated patient

Humidification
The normal function of the upper respiratory tract in humidifying the inspired air must be replaced to prevent desiccation of the mucous

membrane and crusting of secretions. This is most conveniently performed by using a heat and moisture exchanger.

Removal of secretions
Effective coughing is not possible with an intubated larynx and secretions must be removed by suction combined with physiotherapy. Passing a suction catheter must be undertaken as a sterile procedure. The attendants' hands are the greatest source of infection for the intubated patient.

Removal of endotracheal tube

Equipment
This is as for intubation with the addition of a suitable oxygen mask if one is to be used post-extubation.

Procedure
1. Use suction to clear the pharynx, preferably under direct vision using the laryngoscope
2. Deflate the cuff
3. Pass a suction catheter through the tube and withdraw the tube with the suction on. This should be done smoothly and without hesitation
4. Observe the patient's breathing carefully. Repeat aspiration of pharynx if necessary.

43. PHYSIOTHERAPY

There is no doubt that certain patients with respiratory illness are helped by physiotherapy, but many forms of physical therapy are still being evaluated and other time-honoured techniques are now considered ineffective.

OBJECTIVES

Clearance of sputum

Patients with large amounts of sputum as in bronchiectasis, chronic bronchitis or cystic fibrosis may be helped by one or a combination of the following methods.
— Postural drainage
— Forced expiratory technique ('huffing'), in which the patient is encouraged to exhale forcibly through an open mouth
— Forced expiratory technique combined with self compression of the chest wall.
— Percussion and vibration techniques are still widely used although they may be less effective than either of the preceding two methods.
These techniques are commonly combined with bronchodilator therapy.

'Prophylactic'

To prevent retention of sputum in patients with chronic bronchitis whose normal cough is impaired or inhibited after abdominal or thoracic surgery or because of chest wall pain (as from rib fractures).

Mobilisation

Encouragement, advice and assistance from an enthusiastic physiotherapist may speed return to full activity after a severe respiratory illness.

Rehabilitation

Progressive and controlled physical exercise in the form of walking, climbing steps or arm and trunk exercise has been shown to help some patients with chronic respiratory disability (see Chapter 29). Its value may be, in large part, in restoring confidence rather than improving lung function.

Respiratory muscle 'training' in which a patient breaths against a progressively increasing inspiratory resistance has been claimed to improve the performance of respiratory muscles. It has mainly been used during recovery from a recent illness, after a period of assisted ventilation, or after surgery involving the chest wall.

Note: *Nasopharyngeal and oral suction in the conscious patient should never be requested as it is uncomfortable, unsafe and ineffective.*

VALUE OF PHYSIOTHERAPY

Physiotherapy is, in our opinion, of *no proven value* in:
— Lobar pneumonia (in patients without pre-existing lung disease)
— Pulmonary oedema
— Pleural effusion
— Pulmonary embolism
— Aspiration of blood, vomit or gastric contents
— Respiratory failure due to respiratory muscle weakness
— Asthma.

We are not convinced that breathing exercises and relaxation for the emotionally distressed patient, or the patient who 'hyperventilates' is of therapeutic value other than by improving confidence and insight.

Before requesting physiotherapy, consider:
— *In the acutely ill patient* with failure to clear sputum:
  a. Is the patient conscious? Physiotherapy is of no value in the unconscious
  b. Is the patient already being encouraged to cough at regular intervals?
  c. Is the patient receiving other appropriate treatment for airflow obstruction, such as bronchodilators?
— *In the chronically ill patient* with failure to clear sputum:
  a. Is there a partner or relative at home? Postural drainage procedures are usually more effective when assisted by another person. 'Huffing' offers an alternative approach for the single patient
  b. Is appropriate treatment for airways obstruction being used? Many patients with chronic bronchitis, cystic fibrosis or bronchiectasis have some reversibility of airflow obstruction

— *For rehabilitation*:
  a. Has the patient received advice on regular activity or exercise? Progressively increasing physical exercise may be of value, and is often best explained and supervised in the early stages by a physiotherapist
  b. Respiratory muscle training is probably best achieved by gradual increases in activity and exercise but inspiratory muscle training may be of value for bed-bound patients.

INDEX

Abdominal pain, cystic fibrosis, 119
Abram's needle, pleural biopsy, 54–55
Abscess, lung, 89–92
  causes, 89–90
  investigations, 90–91
  treatment, 91–92
Acid-base balance, 44
  abnormalities, 45–46
Acidosis, renal failure, 4
  metabolic, 45
  respiratory, 45
Actinomycosis, 94
Acute bronchitis, 151–152
Air aspiration
  pneumothorax, 130–132
  underwater seal, pneumothorax, 130–131
Air bubbling persistence, pneumothorax, 132
Airway resistance (Raw), 40
Albumin, technetium-labelled, perfusion
      scans, 47–48
Alpha 1 antitrypsin deficiency, emphysema,
      148, 149
Alveolar cell carcinoma, 179
Alveolar gas volume, 38
Alveolitis, 182–186, 223
  see also Cryptogenic fibrosing alveolitis;
      Extrinsic allergic alveolitis
Aminophylline
  dosage, 169
  overdosage dangers, 169–170
Amoebiasis, 10
Anaemia
  blood oxygen levels, 3
  lung function, 41
Anaesthetics, local, nebulisation, 235
Analgesics, asthma precipitation, 201
Anchovy paste sputum, 10
Angiography, pulmonary, 33
  pulmonary hypertension, 80
  thrombo-embolism, 125
Angiotensin, serum levels, sarcoidosis, 188
Antibiotic therapy
  chronic bronchitis, 151
  pneumonia, 85–7
Antibiotics, nebulisation, 235
Anticoagulants, thromboembolic pulmonary
      hyertension, 81
Antinuclear factor, 224
  cryptogenic fibrosing alveolitis, 184–185

pleural effusion, 140
pulmonary hypertension, 80
Antituberculous drugs
  dosages, 102
  side-effects, 103
Aorta
  pain, 19
  traumatic rupture, 198–199
Apneustic respiration, 147
Apnoea, 147
Arterial blood
  gas analysis, 43–46
  chest injuries, 195
  hypoventilation, 145
  pulmonary hypertension, 80
  severe asthma, 168
  thrombo-embolism, 125
  pH, 44, 45–46
  sampling techniques, 43–44
Artificial ventilation
  chest injuries, 192, 196
  respiratory failure, 69, 73, 76
Asbestos
  bronchial carcinoma, 174, 211
  mesothelioma induction, 181, 211
  related diseases, 211
Asbestosis, 183, 211
Ascitic fluid, pleural effusion, 139
Aspergillosis, 94
  broncho-pulmonary, allergic, 59, 60,
      171–172
Aspergillus fumigatus, 59, 60, 84, 171–172, 191
  in cystic fibrosis, 117
Asthma, 156–172
  airflow obstruction, 158
  provocation, 159
  causes, 159–161
  diagnosis, 156–159
    histamine/methacholine inhalation, 159
    history alone, 156
    investigations, 158–159
  differential diagnosis, 162
  drug-induced, 201–2
  family history, 160
  investigation, 161–162
  lung function, 41
  management, 162–167
  occupational, 60, 171, 206–209
    agent identification, 208–209

Asthma (*Cont'd*)
  bronchial challenge tests, 209
  causes, 207
  compensation, 209
  diagnostic sequence, 207–209
  investigations, 207–209
  management and prognosis, 209
  precipitating (trigger) factors, 160–161
  predisposing factors, 159–160
  prophylactic agents, 163–164, 166
  severe acute, 167–170
    investigations, 168
    signs, 168
    treatment, 169–170
  treatment, 169–170
Atmospheric pollution, chronic bronchitis, 148
Atopy
  asthma predisposition, 159–160
  skin tests, 59–60
Azoospermia, cystic fibrosis, 117

Bacterial infections, 94
Barium swallow, 31
  gastro-oesophageal reflux, 21–22
BCG immunisation, 109
Beta blocking agents, asthma precipitation, 201
Bicarbonate, arterial blood levels, 44
Biopsy, 52–53
  alveolitis, 185
  immunodeficiency diseases, 97
  percutaneous, 52
    immunodeficiency diseases, 97
  pleural, 54–55, 139
    bronchial carcinoma, 175–176
  pre-biopsy preparation, 97
  sarcoidosis, 188–189
  surgical (open), 52
    immunodeficiency diseases, 97
    pulmonary hypertension, 80
  transbronchial, 51, 52
  see also various types
Bird fancier's lung, 184, 185, 212
Black sputum, 10
Blood count, asthma, 161
Breathlessness,
  associated symptoms, 5–6
  cardiac dysfunction signs, 6–7
  causes 3–4
  clinical examination, 6–7
  history, 4–6
  investigations, 7
  patient assessment, 4–7
  severe, 153–155
    drug therapy, 155
    psychosocial support, 155
  severity, 4
  speed of onset, 4–5
  timing, 5
Bronchial adenoma, 180
Bronchial carcinoma, 173–179
  asbestos, 174, 211

  cell types, 176
  high risk groups, 174
  investigations, 175–176
  management, 176–179
  metastases, 175, 176
  palliative treatment, 178–179
  small (oat) cell, 176, 178–179
  surgical resection, indications, 176–177
  symptoms and signs, 173–174
Bronchiectasis, 110–114, 115, 183, 224
  associated systemic disorders, 111
  causes, 111
  cystic fibrosis, 115
  diagnosis, 110–113
  investigations, 112–113
  management, 113–114
  resection, 114
  severity assessment, 113
Bronchitis
  ulcerative colitis association, 11
  see also Acute bronchitis; Chronic bronchitis
Broncho-alveolar carcinoma, 179
Broncho-alveolar lavage, alveolitis, 51, 185
Bronchodilators
  asthma, 163
  bronchiectasis, 114
  chronic bronchitis, 150
  cystic fibrosis, 118
  nebulisation, 235
Bronchography, 34
  allergic aspergillosis, 172
  bronchiectasis, 112
  cough, 12
  haemoptysis, 17
Broncho-pleural fistula, empyema, 90
Bronchoscopy, 49–51
  bronchial carcinoma, 175
  bronchiectasis, 112
  cough, 12
  haemoptysis, 17
  immunodeficiency diseases, 96–97
  lung abscess, 91
  segmental or lobar shadowing, 218
  tuberculosis, 101
  see also Fibreoptic bronchoscopy, Rigid
    bronchoscopy
Bronchus, ruptured, 198

'Café-coronary', 120, 121
Calcium, serum levels, sarcoidosis, 188
  see also Hypercalcaemia
Candidiasis
  Pulmonary, 94
  oral, 163
Caplan's syndrome, 210
Carbon dioxide gas transfer (TLCO), 38–39
  interpretation, 39
Carboxyhaemoglobin, 39
Carcinoma,
  metastasis, 180
  bronchoalveolar, 179
  see also Bronchial carcinoma

Cardiac catheterisation, pulmonary
    hypertension, 80
Cardiac injuries, 199
Cardiac pain, 19
Cardiac tamponade, 199
Cephalosporins, pneumonia, 86
Chemotherapy, small (oat) cell carcinoma,
    178–179
Chest pain *see* Pain
Chest wall disease, 144
  lung function, 41
Chest wall injuries, 194
Chest X-ray
  abnormal, 216–226
  acute thrombo-embolism, 124–125
  alveolitis, 182, 184
  anterior-posterior (AP) view, 29
  apical lordotic view, 30
  asbestosis, 211
  asthma, 161
  bronchial carcinoma, 175
  bronchiectasis, 112
  chest injuries, 197
  chest pain, 21
  chronic bronchitis, 149
  cystic fibrosis, 116
  diffuse lung shadowing, 222–224
  drug induced lung disease, 202–204
  examination, 31–32
  haemoptysis, 16
  impaired defences, 95
  inhaled foreign body, 121
  lateral film, 29
  lobar shadowing, 216–218
  lung abscess, 90
  lung tumours, 175
  oblique projections, 30
  over-exposed views, 30
  'overpenetrated' views, 30
  pleural effusion, 136
  pneumoconiosis, 210
  pneumonia, 83
  pneumothorax, 128
  pre-operative, 32
  pulmonary eosinophilia, 213–215
  pulmonary hypertension, 78
  sarcoidosis, 187–188
  segmental shadowing, 216–218
  severe asthma, 168
  solitary lung mass, 218–220
  standard, 29
  thromboembolism, 124
  tuberculosis, 101
Cheyne-Stokes respiration, 147
Chronic bronchitis, 148–155
  assessment, 153–155
  complications, 151–152
  differential diagnosis, 150
  investigations, 149
  lung function, 41
  obstructive, 41
  occupational causes, 148
  respiratory failure, 71, 74,
    76

symptoms and signs, 149
  treatment, 150–151
Cigarette smoking
  bronchial carcinoma, 173, 174
  chronic bronchitis, 148
Cirrhosis, cystic fibrosis, 117
Clotting screen, haemoptysis, 16
Coal worker's pneumoconiosis, 210
Coeliac disease, 190
Computed tomography, 33
  lung cancer, 177
  mediastinal disease, 22
  solitary lung mass, 219
Consciousness, coughing ability effects, 8
Contusion, pulmonary, 196
Cor pulmonale, chronic bronchitis, 153
Corridor walking distance test, 40
Cough
  clinical assessment, 9–12
  complications, 12
  dry, causes, 9
  history, 11
  investigations, 11–12
  normal mechanisms, 8
  treatment, 13
CREST syndrome, pulmonary hypertension,
    79
Crohn's disease, 190
Cryptococcosis, 94
Cryptogenic fibrosing alveolitis, 182–186, 223
  dermatomyositis, 184
  investigations, 184–185
  rheumatoid arthritis, 184
  treatment, 186
Cycle ergometer exercise test, 42
Cystic fibrosis, 111, 115–119
  assessment, 117
  genetic counselling, 119
  management, 117–119
  physical examination and diagnosis,
    115–116
  respiratory features and complications, 116
  respiratory exacerbation, 118–119
  symptoms, 115
Cytomegalovirus infections, 95

Delayed reactions, atopy skin tests, 59
Dermatomyositis, cryptogenic fibrosing
    alveolitis, 184
Diabetes mellitus, cystic fibrosis, 117
Diabetic acidosis, 3–4
Diaphragm
  paralysis, 220–21
  raised, 220
  ruptured, 198
Diuretics, chronic hypoxia, 71
Doxopram, respiratory failure, 73
Drill (high speed trephine) biopsy, 52
Drug reactions, 94
Drugs
  lung disease induction, 201–204, 223
  nebulisation, 234–235

Echocardiogram, pulmonary hypertension, 78
Edinburgh oxygen mask, 230
Electrocardiogram
  acute thrombo-embolism, 125
  chest pain, 21
  haemoptysis, 16
  hypoventilation, 145
  pulmonary hypertension, 78
  severe asthma, 168
Embolectomy, surgical, 127
Embolism, pulmonary
  isotope scans, 48
  lung function, 41
  massive, 124
    thrombolytic therapy, 126–127
  see also Thrombo-embolism, acute
Emphysema, 148–155
  assessment, 153–155
  complications, 151–152
  lung function, 41
  'respiratory cripples', 153–155
  surgical, 193–194
    transtracheal aspiration, 58
Empyema, 88
  broncho-pleural fistula, 90
  in pneumonia, 88
  management, 141–143
  pleural effusion, 138
  tuberculous, pleural calcification, 222
Endotracheal intubation, 239–242
  equipment, 239–240
  indications, 239
  problems and complications, 241
  technique, 240–41
  tube removal, 242
Eosinophilia, pulmonary, 183, 213
  aspergillosis-associated, 171
  in asthma, 213
  cryptogenic, 213–214
  drug induced, 203
  parasitic, 214
  vasculitis, 214
Erythema nodosum, 187, 190
  management, 191
Erythrophoresis, chronic hypoxia, 70–71
ESR, tuberculosis, 100
Ethambutol
  adverse effects, 103
  dosage, 102
Exercise tolerance, tests, 40, 42
Extrinsic allergic alveolitis, 182–186, 223, 224.
  differential diagnosis, 183–184
  investigations, 184–185
  occupational, 212
  treatment, 186
Exudate, pleural effusion, 138

Farmer's lung, 184, 185, 212
Fibreoptic bronchoscopy, 49–51
  indications, 49–50
  patient preparation, 50
  procedures, 50–51

Fibrosis, pulmonary
  diffuse, 211
  lung function, 41
  sarcoidosis, 190
Fibrothorax, 197
Finger clubbing,
  alveolitis, 184
  bronchial carcinoma, 174
Flail chest, 193, 195
Flow volume loop (FV curve), 40
Fluoroscopy, diaphragmatic function, 31
Forced expiratory volume (FEV1), 36–38
  normal values, 37
Foreign bodies, inhaled, 120–122, 192
  management, 121–122
Functional residual volume (FRV), lung,
  39–40
Fungal infections, 94–95
  see also individual diseases

Gamma imaging, 48
Gasping respiration, 147
Gastro-oesophageal reflux, 19
  barium swallow, 21–22
Genetic counselling, cystic fibrosis, 119
Goodpasture's syndrome, 16, 223
Great vessels, penetrating injuries, 199
Grey sputum, 10
Gullain-Barré syndrome, 71

Haemopericardium, 199
Haemophilus influenzae
  cystic fibrosis, 117
  chronic bronchitis, 152
Haemopneumothorax, 128
Haemoptysis, 14–18
  causes and symptoms, 14–15
  clinical assessment, 14–17
  cystic fibrosis, 119
  emergency treatment, 17–18
  examination, 15
  investigations, 16–17
  management, 17–18
Haemorrhage
  alveolar, 223
  chest injuries, 193, 194
  intrapleural, chest injuries, 196–197
  pulmonary, 94
Haemothorax, 197
  pleural calcification, 222
Heaf test, 61–62
  results grading, 62
Heart-lung transplantation, 81
Heimlich (flutter) valve, pneumothorax, 131
Heimlich manoeuvre, 'café-coronary', 121
Heparin, pulmonary embolism, 126
Herpes virus infections, 95
Hiatus hernia, 90
Hilar lymph node enlargement, 180, 187, 223
Hodgkin's disease, 180, 225–226

Humidifier fever, 212
Hypercalcaemia, sarcoidosis, 188, 191
Hypercapnia,
  with acute hypoxia, 71–74
  Chest wall, neurovascular disease, 145
  chronic bronchitis, 152
  with chronic hypoxia, 74–76
Hypersensitivity reactions, asthma, 201–202
Hypertension, pulmonary, 77–81
  associated disorders, 77
  cause diagnosis, 79
  diagnosis, 78
  hypoxia, 69
  investigations, 78, 80
  management, 81
  symptoms and signs, 78
  thromboembolic, 79, 81
Hyperthyroidism, breathlessness, 3
Hyperventilation, 4
  central neurogenic, 147
  physiotherapy, 244
Hypoventilation, 144–147
  investigation, 145–146
  sleep, 146–147
Hypoxia, acute, 68–69
  with hypercapnia, 71–74
    associated disorders, 71–72
    management, 72–74
Hypoxia, chronic, 69–76
  with hypercapnia, 74–76
    associated disorders, 74
    management, 75–76

Immotile cilia syndrome, 112
Immunodeficiency, respiratory disorders,
    93–98
Immunoglobulin E antibodies,
    allergen-induced, 59, 160, 209
Imotest, 62
Indomethacin, pleural pain relief, 85
Infarction, pulmonary, 94
  pleural effusion, 140
Infertility, cystic fibrosis, 117
Injuries, chest, 192–200
  embedded objects, 193, 197
  initial assessment, 192–194
  management, 194–200
    initial, 192–194
  penetrating, 197
Inspiratory crackles,
  early, 23–24, 25
  late, 24–25
Intercostal drains, 236–238
  chest injury, 194, 197
  emphysema, 143
  indications, 236
  insertion sites, 236
  insertion technique, 236–238
  pleural effusion, 140
  pneumothorax, 130
  removal, 238
  suction and, 238

Intestinal obstruction, cystic fibrosis, 119
Intracardiac shunts, 44
IPPB, severe breathlessness, 155
Irradiation
  in lung cancer, 178
  pulmonary effects, 94
  in superior vena cava obstruction, 179
Isoniazid
  adverse effects, 103
  dosage, 102
Isotope lung scans, 47–48
  haemoptysis, 17
  safety, 48
  thrombo-embolism, 125

Krypton-81, lung scans, 47
Kveim test, sarcoidosis, 189–190, 224

Laryngoscopy, indirect, cough, 12
Left ventricular failure, 183
  chest X-ray, 223
Legionella infection, 84
Leukaemia, 94
Lung
  diffusing capacity, 38–9
  functional residual volume, 39–40
  over-inflation, 24
  residual volume (RV), 38, 39–40
  total lung capacity, 39–40
Lung function tests, 35–42
  pulmonary hypertension, 80
  sarcoidosis, 190
Lung mass, solitary, 218–220
Lupus syndrome
  drug-induced, 204
  SLE and pleural effusion, 135
Lymph nodes,
  enlargement, sarcoidosis, 187–188
  intrathoracic, enlargement, 187, 223
  tuberculosis, 108
Lymphadenitis, tuberculous, 190
Lymphoma, 94
  intrathoracic, 180
  superior vena cava obstruction, 179

Malabsorption, cystic fibrosis, 119
Malt worker's lung, 212
Mantoux test, 61
MC oxygen mask, 228
'Meconium ileus equivalent', cystic fibrosis,
    117
Mediastinal lymph nodes, pain, 20
Mediastinal masses, 225–226
Mediastinitis, superior vena cava obstruction,
    179
Mediastinoscopy
  bronchial carcinoma, 176
  tuberculosis, 101

Mediastinotomy, bronchial carcinoma, 174
Meningitis, tuberculous, 108
Mesothelioma
  pleural and peritoneal, 211
  pleural effusion, 135
  primary malignant, 181
Metabolic acidosis, 3, 45
Metabolic alkalosis, 45
Metastases, pulmonary, 94, 180
Micropolyspora faeni, 185
Mitral stenosis, pulmonary hypertension, 79
Monophonic wheeze, 23
Mucoid sputum, 10
Mucolytics
  nebulisation, 233
  chronic bronchitis, 151
Mucormycosis, 95
Mucus plugs, 10
Mushroom worker's lung, 212
Mycetoma, haemoptysis, 191
Mycobacteria, 'atypical', 107
Mycobacterium tuberculosis, 100
  drug resistance, 105–106
  sputum culture, 100
Mycoplasma pneumoniae, 84, 85
  diffuse lung shadowing, 223

Needle aspiration biopsy, 52
  bronchial carcinoma, 176
  lung abscess, 91
  see also Abram's needle; Trucut needle
    biopsy
Nerve root pain, 20
Neuromuscular disease
  lung function, 41
  hypoventilation, 144
Nocardiosis, 94

Obesity, hypoventilation, 145
Occupational lung diseases, 205–12
  asthma, 171, 206
Oedema, pulmonary, 10, 94, 183
  lung function, 41
  alterpneumothorax, 133
Oesophagus
  injuries, 200
  pain, 19
Opacity, circumsribed, pulmonary, 218–220
Opportunist infections, 94–95, 95
Osteoarthropathy, hypertrophic, cystic fibrosis,
    117
  lung cancer, 174
Oxygen therapy, 229–233
  acute hypoxia/hypercapnia, 72–73
  bronchitis and emphysema, 154
  chest injuries, 195
  chronic hypoxia, 70
  chronic hypoxia/hypercapnia, 75–6
  domiciliary, long-term, 232–233
  flow regulators, 230
  gas delivery, 230–31

gas supply, 229–230
  humidification, 231
  indications, 229
  masks, 230–31
  pneumonia, 84–85
  principles, 229
  risks and toxicity, 232
  fever asthma, 169

Pain, chest, 19–22
  examination, 21
  history, 20
    treatment in chest injuries, 194–195
  investigations, 21–22
  sites of origin, 19–20
  treatment, 22
Pancoast syndrome, 173
Pancreas, function tests, cystic fibrosis, 116
Pancreatic steatorrhoea, cystic fibrosis, 117
Parasitic infections, pulmonary eosinophilia,
    214–215
Patient mobilisation, physiotherapy, 243
Peak expiratory flow rate (PEFR), 35–36
Perfusion scans, isotope, 47–48
  pulmonary hypertension, 80
Pericardium, pain, 19
Peripheral nerve disorders, hypoventilation,
    144
Physical training, severe breathlessness, 155
Physiotherapy, 243–245
  objectives, 243–244
  prophylactic, 243
  value, 244–245
Platelet counts, haemoptysis, 16
Pleura
  biopsy, 54–55, 139
    carcinoma, 175
    equipment, 54
    technique, 54
    tuberculosis, 101
  calcification, radiology, 222
  masses, radiology, 221–222
  opacities, 221
  pain, 19, 85
  thickening, radiology, 221
  tumours, 180–181
Pleural aspiration
  bronchial carcinoma, 175–176
  pleural effusion, 136–137
Pleural effusion, 134–143, 219
  asbestos-related, 211
  cause diagnosis, 134–136
  chylous and pseudochylous, 138–139
  diagnostic aspiration, 136–137
  fluid appearances, 137–138
  fluid examination, 137
  intercostal drain site, 234
  investigations, 136–140
  malignant cells, 140
  Pneumonia, 87
  radiology, 136, 221
  surgery, 141

Pleural effusion (*Cont'd*)
  thromboembolism, 125
  treatment, 140–141
Pleural fibrosis, asbestos-related, 211
Pleural plaques, asbestos-related, 211
Pleurectomy, pneumothorax, 133
Pleurodesis
  chemical, pleural effusion, 141
  pneumothorax, 133
Pneumococcal antigen, pneumonia, 84
Pneumoconiosis, 210–211, 224
Pneumocystis carinii, 95
  pneumonia, 84, 183
Pneumonia, 82–88, 183
  antibiotic therapy, 85–87
  causes, 84
  chronic bronchitis, 152
  clinical picture, 82
  investigations, 83
  lobar, 84, 217
  management, 84–88
  necrotising, 90
  physical examination, 82–83
  pleural pain relief, 85
  prolonged fever, 88
  transbronchial aspiration, 56
  treatment
    response assessment, 87
    response failure, 87–88
  unresolved, 88
  'ventilation', 212
  viral, 220
Pneumothorax, 128–132
  air removal, 129–132, 238
    technique, 130–132
  causes, 128
  chest injuries, 192–193, 194
  diagnosis, 128
  differential diagnosis, 129
  expiration X-rays, 30–31
  intercostal tube
    site, 234
    suction, 236
  lung expansion failure, 132
  management, 129–133
    problems, 132–133
  tension, 192–193
Polycythaemia
  hypoventilation, 146
  secondary, hypoxia, 69
Polyphonic wheeze, 23
Prednisolone, pulmonary eosinophilia, 172
  asthma, 164, 167, 169
  pneumonia, 86
Pseudomonas aeruginosa, cystic fibrosis, 115
Pulmonary artery catheterisation, pulmonary
    hypertension, 78
Pulmonary reactions, diffuse
  drug-induced, 202–204
  fibrosis 203–204
Pulsus paradoxus, 199
Pus, pleural effusion, 138, 141–143
  see also Empyema
Pyrazinamide

  adverse effects, 103
  dosage, 102

Radiotherapy, bronchial carcinoma, 178
Raynaud's phenomenon, systemic sclerosis,
    184
Rehabilitation, physiotherapy, 244
Rehydration, pneumonia, 85
Renal tuberculosis, 108
Residual volume (RV), lung, 39–40
Respiration
  abnormal patterns, 147
  anaerobic, 3
  noisy, 24
Respiratory acidosis, 45
Respiratory alkalosis, 45
Respiratory centres, disease, hypoventilation,
    144
'Respiratory cripples', bronchitis and
    emphysema, 153–155
Respiratory defences, impaired, 93–98
  diagnosis, 93–98
  management of infections, 95–98
Respiratory failure, 67–76
  acute hypoxic, 68–69
    causes, 68
    management, 68–69
  chronic bronchitis, 152–153
  chronic hypoxic, 69–71
    causes, 69
    investigations, 70
    management, 70–71
  nocturnal, 76
  symptoms and signs, 67
  types, 67
Respiratory function tests, 35–42
  alveolitis, 182
  chronic bronchitis, 149
  cystic fibrosis, 117
  lung cancer, 177
  pulmonary hypertension, 80
  sarcoidosis, 190
Respiratory movements, measurement,
    hypoventilation, 145–146
Rheumatoid arthritis, cryptogenic fibrosing
    alveolitis association, 184
Rheumatoid factor
  cryptogenic fibrosing alveolitis, 184–185
    184–185
  diffuse lung shadowing, 224
  pleural effusion, 140
  pulmonary hypertension, 80
Ribs
  fractures, 194
  pain, 20
Rifampicin
  adverse effects, 103
  dosage, 102
Right ventricular hypertrophy
  chronic bronchitis, 153
  pulmonary hypertension, 78
Rigid bronchoscopy

Rigid bronchoscopy (Cont'd)
    indications, 51
    inhaled foreign body, 122
Rusty sputum, 10

Salicylate poisoning, breathlessness, 3
Saliva, differentiation from sputum, 10, 11
Sarcoidosis, 184, 187–191, 222, 223, 224
    course and prognosis, 190–191
    diagnosis, 187–188
    extra-thoracic, management, 189, 191
    hypercalcaemia, 188, 191
    investigations, 185–190
    management, 191
    natural history, 190–191
    ocular, 189, 191
    tissue biopsies, 188–189
Serum enzymes, thrombo-embolism, 125
Shock, chest injuries, 193
Shock lung, 94, 183
Silicosis, 210–211
Skin tests
    asthma, 162
    atopy, 59–60
    extrinsic alveolitis, 185
    tuberculin, 61–63
Solid tissue expectoration, 10
Spirometry, 36–38
Sputum, 9–11
    appearances, 10–11
    clearance, 243
    cultures
    bronchiestasis, 113
    chronic bronchitis, 152
    lung abscess, 91
    pneumonia, 83, 87
    tuberculosis, 100
    cystic fibrosis, 115, 117
    cytological examination, 12
        bronchial carcinoma, 175
    differentiation from saliva, 10, 11
    large quantities, causes, 11
    smell, 11
    stained smears, tuberculosis, 100
    types, 10
    see also various types
Staphylococcus pyogenes, 84, 85
    cystic fibrosis, 115
    lung abscess, 89
    pneumonia, 84, 85, 87
Status asthmaticus, 168
Steatorrhoea, pancreatic, cystic fibrosis, 117
Sternum, fractures, 194
Stiff lungs, 24–25
Streptococcus pneumoniae,
    chronic bronchitis, 152
    pneumonia, 84, 85
Streptokinase
    massive pulmonary embolism, 126–127
    contraindictions, 127
Superior vena cava obstruction, 179
Sweat test, cystic fibrosis, 112, 115–116

Systemic sclerosis, Raynaud's phenomenon,
    184

Tartrazine dyes, asthma induction, 192
Technetium-99
    albumin labelling, perfusion scans, 47–48
    DTPA chelated, lung scans, 47
Thermoactinomvces vulgaris, 185
Thoracoscopy, pleural effusion, 139
Thoracotomy
    chest injuries, 197–199
    pleural effusion, 140
Thrombo-embolism; acute, 123–127
    investigations, 124–125
    physical signs, 124
    risk factors, 123
    symptoms, 123–124
    treatment, 126–127
Thrombolytic therapy
    complications and risks, 127
    pulmonary embolism, 126–127
Tine tuberculin test, 62
Tomography, 32–33, 217
    see also Computed tomography
Toxoplasmosis, 95
Tracheitis, 19
Tracheostomy, indications, chest injuries, 196
Transbronchial aspiration, 56–58
    complications, 58
    contraindications, 56
    immunodeficiency diseases, 96
    indications, 56
    lung abscess, 91
    technique, 56–58
Transbronchial biopsy
    alveolitis, 185
    immunodeficiency diseases, 97
    sarcoidosis, 189
    technique, 52
Transudate, pleural effusion, 138
Treadmil exercise test, 42
Trephine (drill) biopsy, 52
Trucut needle biopsy, 52
    pleura, 54
Tuberculin test, 61–63, 101
    clinical value, 63
    significance, 62–63
Tuberculosis, 99–109, 183, 226
    chemoprophylaxis, 107
    contacts, 104, 106
        examination, 106
        tuberculin test, 63
    extrathoracic, 108
    follow-up, 106
    infection spread control, 104, 106
    investigations, 100–101
    management, 102–109
    place of treatment, 104
    reactivation prevention, 107
    treatment
        non-compliance, 104–105
        observation, 105

Tuberculosis (*Cont'd*)
   response failure, 105–106
   supervision, 104–105

Ulcerative colitis, 190
Ultrasound examination, 34
Urine, red blood cells, haemoptysis, 16
Urokinase, massive pulmonary embolism,
     126–127

Vasculitis, systemic, 214
Vasodilators, pulmonary hypertension, 81
Venesection, chronic hypoxia, 70–71
Venography, lower limb, thrombo-embolism, 125
Ventilation, assisted
  acute respiratory failure, 74
  chest injuries, 196
  chronic respiratory failure, 76
'Ventilation pneumonia', 212

Ventilation scans, isotope, 47–48
  pulmonary hypertension, 80
Venturi masks, 230
Virus diseases, 95
Vital capacity, forced (FVC), 36–38
  normal values, 38
  stiff lungs, 24
Vitalography, 36–38

Warfarin, pulmonary embolism, 126
Watery sputum, 10
Weals, skin tests, 59
Wheezes, 23

Xenon-133, lung scans, 47

Yellow nail syndrome, 111